# of Ultrasound in Obstetrics, Gynecology and Infertility

Step by Step

Tips and Tricks
of Ultrasound in Obstetrics,
Gynecology and Infertility

Kuldeep Singh

MBBS FAUI FICMCH
Consultant Ultrasonologist
Special Interest in Obstetric Sonology
in Detailed Anomaly Scanning and
Color Doppler for Management and Gynecological Scanning
Conducts FOGSI recognised ultrasound training courses in
Obstetrics, Gynecology and Infertility
(Basics, Color Doppler, 3D and Line 3D)
Ultrasound training division: 011-9212117174
Dr Kuldeep's Ultrasound and Color Doppler Clinic
D-115, East of Kailash, New Delhi 110065 (India)
Phones: 011-26441720, 26233342 Mobile: 98111 96613
singhdrkuldeep@rediffmail.com

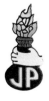

JAYPEE BROTHERS
MEDICAL PUBLISHERS (P) LTD
New Delhi

Published by

Jitendar P Vij

Jaypee Brothers Medical Publishers (P) Ltd

EMCA House, 23/23B Ansari Road, Daryaganj **New Delhi** 110 002, India
Phones: +91-11-23272143, +91-11-23272703, +91-11-23282021,
+91-11-23245672   Fax: +91-11-23276490, +91-11-23245683
e-mail: jaypee@jaypeebrothers.com
Visit our web site: www.jaypeebrothers.com

Branches

- 202 Batavia Chambers, 8 Kumara Krupa Road, Kumara Park East
  Bangalore 560 001, Phones: +91-80-22285971, +91-80-22382956,
  +91-80-30614073 Tele Fax : +91-80-22281761
  e-mail: jaypeebc@bgl.vsnl.net.in

- 282 IIIrd Floor, Khaleel Shirazi Estate, Fountain Plaza, Pantheon Road
  Chennai 600 008, Phones: +91-44-28262665, +91-44-28269897
  Fax: +91-44-28262331 e-mail: jpmedpub@md3.vsnl.net.in

- 4-2-1067/1-3, Ist Floor, Balaji Building, Ramkote Cross Road,
  Hyderabad 500 095, Phones: +91-40-55610020, +91-40-24758498
  Fax: +91-40-24758499
  e-mail: jpmedpub@rediffmail.com

- 1A Indian Mirror Street, Wellington Square, **Kolkata** 700 013
  Phone: +91-33-22451926 Fax: +91-33-22456075
  e-mail: jpbcal@cal.vsnl.net.in

- 106 Amit Industrial Estate, 61 Dr SS Rao Road, Near MGM Hospital
  Parel, **Mumbai** 400 012 Phones: +91-22-24124863,
  +91-22-24104532, +91-22-30926896   Fax: +91-22-24160828
  e-mail: jpmedpub@bom7.vsnl.net.in

***Step by Step Tips and Tricks of Ultrasound in
Obstetrics, Gynecology and Infertility***

First Edition: **2005**

ISBN 81-8061-463-8

Typeset at JPBMP typesetting unit

Printed at   Paras Offset Pvt. Ltd., C-176, Naraina Industrial Area, Phase-1, New Delhi 110028

This book is dedicated
to my parents
Mrs Yoginder Kaur
Mr KJ Singh
who are with God

Preface

So much is dependent on the operator using the machine that one needs to be aware of the small mistakes we can and we all make during our practice.

This book has been made according to the daily practical routines, problems and discrepancies we all face.

It is going to be a handy book for anybody using this diagnostic modality.

Kuldeep Singh

Acknowledgements

This book would never have been possible without the help of my seniors and well wishers who have stood by me and given me the confidence and the driving force to accomplish these feats. Special mention for Dr Narendra Malhotra (Agra), Dr Jaideep Malhotra (Agra), Dr PK Shah (Mumbai), Dr Bhupendra Ahuja (Agra), Dr S Suresh (Chennai), Dr Satpal Gupta and Dr Kamal Gupta (Jalandhar), Dr Anita Sharma (Jalandhar), Dr Nutan Jain (Muzaffarnagar), Dr AS Saini (Amritsar), Dr Mala Arora (Faridabad) and Dr Mitra Saxena (Rewari).

Special thanks to my teacher Dr Ashok Khurana and my seniors in Delhi, Dr RN Bagga, Dr Varun Duggal, Dr Renu Caprihan, Dr Deepak Chawla and Dr Manju Virmani.

The patience that my family has shown in bearing my absence from their time is phenomenal. Nishu K Singh my wife and my children Suzi, Jaanvi Sana Chhabra and Ramanjeet Singh, thank you very much for sparing me on those late evenings and Sundays.

Mrs Mansi Basu thanks to you for all the help in typing. Thanks to Mr JP Vij, Chairman and Managing Director, Jaypee Brothers Medical Publishers (P) Ltd, for providing these platforms and to Mr Tarun Duneja, General Manager (Publishing), Mr PS Ghuman, Senior Production Manager and Mrs Yashu Kapoor for the finer details.

Contents

1. First Personal Contact with Your Machine *1*

2. Interaction with the Patient
   and Transducer Application
   and Movements *11*

3. Pregnancy with a Normal First
   Trimester (04-12 Weeks) *18*

4. Interaction with the Pregnancy
   and Fetus *26*

5. Abnormal Intrauterine Gestational Sac *41*

6. Abnormal Pregnancy: First Trimester *48*

7. First Trimester *61*

8. Normal Second Trimester: Extra-Fetal *65*

9. Normal Second Trimester: Fetal Evaluation *75*

10. Extra-Fetal Variations: Second Trimester *85*

11. Abnormal Second Trimester:
    Fetal Evaluation *94*

12. Wellbeing in the Third Trimester *111*

13. Fetal Wellbeing by Biophysical Scoring
    and Color Doppler Studies *122*

14. Summary of Obstetric Scanning *132*

15. Normal Female Pelvis *134*

16. Uterine Disorders *143*

17. Ovarian Disorders *159*

18. **Miscellaneous Disorders of Female Pelvis ......** *169*

19. **Ultrasound, Color Doppler and
3D Ultrasound for Assessment of
an Infertile Female ....** *175*

Appendices

1. *Normal Values ....* *190*

2. *Measurement Methodology ....* *194*

3. *Reporting ....* *197*

4. *Schematic Analysis for Fetal Anomalies ....* *201*

5. *Fetal Abnormalities in Trisomy
21, 18 and 13 ....* *204*

6. *Fetal Abnormalities in Triploidy and
Turner's Syndrome ....* *207*

7. *Fetal Abnormalities in Maternal Infections ....* *209*

Index *211*

First Personal Contact with Your Machine

The moment you enter the room what all do you see:
1. Ultrasound machine.
2. An external device to record the images you are going to get on the screen.
3. UPS, CVT or a stabilizer to give constant electric supply.

Ultrasound Machine

The machine basically consists of
1. Monitor
   a. Screen for viewing the ultrasound pictures
   b. Knobs for increasing or decreasing the contrast and brightness
2. Transducers
   a. Transabdominal transducer (3-5 MHz)
   b. Transvaginal/transrectal transducer (5-8 MHz)
      One can have a single port in which you can interchange the probes or you can have dual ports one for each of them. There is always a place for the jelly bottle in the transducer stand.
3. Front panel with all knobs
   a. On/off switch. Be very gentle while switching on or off the machine.
   b. Freeze button. Can be operated on the front panel or by a foot switch.
   c. New patient. Can start fresh and operate the submenu one wants to use. Fill in the name of the patient and other information like LMP, etc. on the board (Fig. 1.1).
   d. B: Denotes a single 2D image on the screen (Fig. 1.2).
   e. B+B: Denotes two 2D images on the screen (Fig. 1.3).
   f. B+M: Denotes a single 2D image and M-mode tracing on the screen (Fig. 1.4).
   g. M: Denotes only M-mode tracing on the screen (Fig. 1.5).

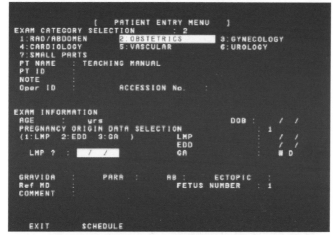

Fig. 1.1: This is the page you see on the screen when your machine is on. Feed the patients name, number and ID for future references. Fill in the details of LMP, EDD, etc. for your calculations

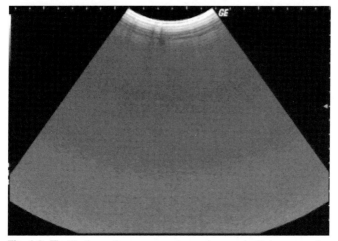

Fig. 1.2: That is the pattern you see to produce a single image on the screen. The region of interest can be zoomed (enlarged) accordingly on the screen itself

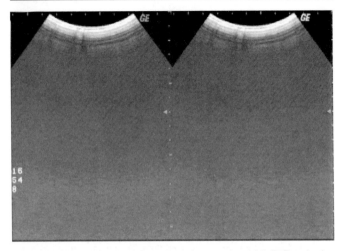

Fig. 1.3: More information can be given when you have this B+B projection on the screen. Respective labeling and measurements can be done accordingly for both the images

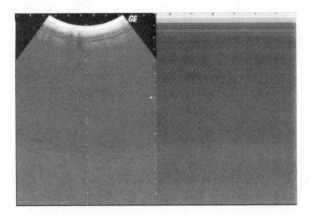

Fig. 1.4: This M-mode is used for recording and calculating heart rate

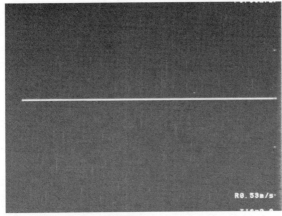

Fig. 1.5: Only M-mode tracing

h. CFM (Fig. 1.6), PD (Fig. 1.7), 3D are knobs for advanced machines.

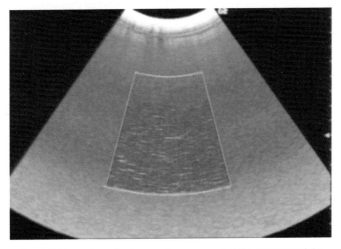

Fig. 1.6: You get a color box on the screen and the intensity of the color can be increased or decreased accordingly

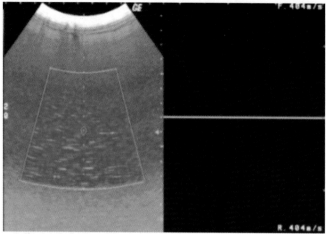

Fig. 1.7: With the color box on you can put a cursor on the blood vessel of interest and get a waveform for further calculations

i. Comment: This is for labeling. The cursor can be moved by a trackball, joystick or a touch screen and you can label the region of interest. One can also use the auto annotations where the complete label is typed within the machine. There is a complete keyboard on the panel usually for typing (Fig. 1.8).

j. Measurement: Press this button and you can get a plus (+) (Fig. 1.9) sign on the screen. Go to one edge of whichever region you are measuring press the SET button and you can go to the other edge. Press set again and you get the measurement in mm or cm on the screen itself (Fig. 1.10). Press SELECT for the next set of measurements (Fig. 1.11).

k. Set: Denotes completion of whichever activity you are doing.

l. Select: Denotes going to the other menu.

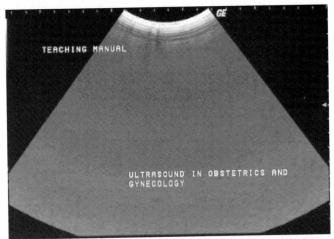

Fig. 1.8: You can label your pictures as it gives more information to the referring doctor. One can start labeling a particular portion and then move the cursor and label at a different location

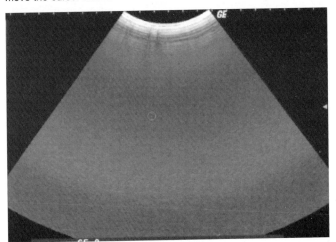

Fig. 1.9: To start measurements press the measurement button and take the marker to one end of whatever you need to measure. Once you localize at that area press the SET button

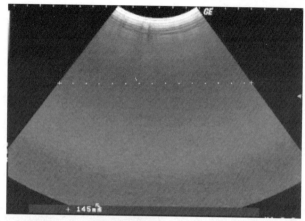

Fig. 1.10: The moment you press the SET button the other marker comes on the screen. Take this marker to the other end of the region you need to measure and press the SET button. You will get the measurement in mm or cm on the screen. The position where this measurement appears can be different for all machines

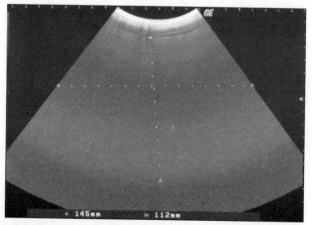

Fig. 1.11: For the next set of measurements press the SELECT button. The cursor again appears. Do the same maneuvering again to get the measurements

m. TGC knobs: Denotes increasing or decreasing the echoes in a particular portion of the screen (Fig. 1.12).

n. Overall gain: Increases/Decreases the overall brightness of the picture (Fig. 1.13).

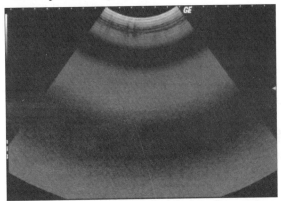

Fig. 1.12: With the TGC knobs one can increase or decrease the intensity of signals in a particular area of the screen. On the screen you get this zebra appearance

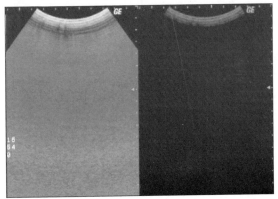

Fig. 1.13: With the overall gain knob one can increase or decrease the intensity of signals on the whole screen. Compare the picture on the left side as it is more bright with the picture on the right which is more dark

o. Read the manual carefully, treat your machine with respect and hold the transducer firmly.

External Device

For printing the pictures you get on the screen one can have the following devices:
1. Camera
2. Thermal paper printing
3. Computer down loading the pictures which you can take out on a printer or a CD/floppy.

For Constant Power Supply

Check with your manufacturer the alternative power supply one can use and secondly to get a constant voltage supply what all can be used.

CHAPTER 2

Interaction with the Patient and Transducer Application and Movements

Make the patient feel comfortable in your company. Talk to them in detail regarding their ailments either in infertility, gynecology or obstetrics. Get a mental frame as to what could be the problem with her symptoms and the examination notes.

Steps for Ultrasound Examination

1. Fill in the patients form with all particulars: Name, Age, Address, Telephone Number and Referral Doctor.
   a. Mention clinical information in your notes. Previous obstetric history consisting of previous pregnancy details if any, Any symptoms in this pregnancy, Any ultrasound done so far in this pregnancy, Last menstrual period and regularity of menstrual cycles, Any other tests done and their reports. Form F (and any other forms) have to be filled up for the PNDT Act as required by the Government laws.
2. Enter patients name and details on the machine.
3. Pour jelly on the patients abdomen or your transducer.
4. Orient yourself as to the right and left of the screen. The left of the transducer and the left of the screen denote right of the patient and vice versa. For any doubts press your finger gently on the edge of the transducer to coordinate position on the screen.
5. To correctly assess when you are keeping the transducer in a transverse position the left of the screen is the patient's right (Fig. 2.1) and vice versa, and when you are keeping the transducer in a longitudinal position the left of the screen is the cranial/superior end of the patient (Fig. 2.2) and vice versa.
6. Assess the full bladder. Urinary bladder should be adequately full (Fig. 2.3) with the portion you want to

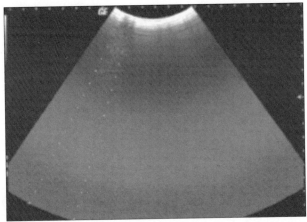

Fig. 2.1: Note the left end of the picture where you get the impression of the finger being pressed. This is a transverse section and this is to the right of the patient

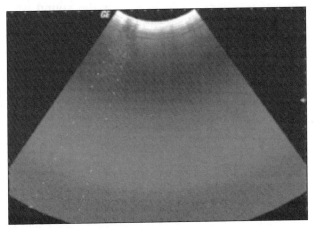

Fig. 2.2: Note the left end of the picture where you get the impression of the finger being pressed. This is the longitudinal section and this is the cranial/superior end of the patient

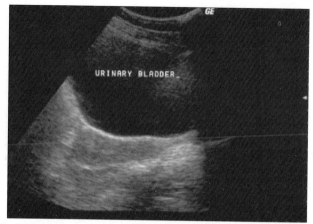

Fig. 2.3: Picture of an adequately full urinary bladder. The uterine fundus should be seen through the urinary bladder window

study should have the bladder for a window rather than bowel which is going to scatter the sound waves. Remember no short cuts, if bladder is partially full (Fig. 2.4) wait for it to fill up and if it is overdistended (Fig. 2.5) tell the patient to void and come back.

7. Start noticing the structures you see behind the bladder and start making an impression as to what you are seeing is normal or not.

8. Don't be in a rush to complete the study. Look very carefully for adjacent structures and try and get a clue from it.

9. For transvaginal scanning the patient is asked to void urine. It should be performed with the same respect for privacy and gentleness, as is with the placement of a speculum. Scanning is performed with the patient supine and with her thighs abducted and knees flexed. Elevation of the buttock may be necessary. The probe should be covered with a condom or sheath containing a small amount of

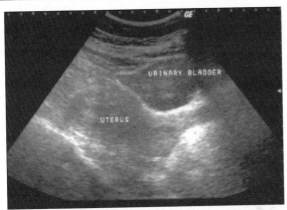

Fig. 2.4: With the portion you want to study should have the bladder for a window rather than bowel which is going to scatter the sound waves. So remember if the bladder is partially full wait for it to fill up. In this picture the bladder is not seen in front of the uterine fundus, it is seen only till the uterine corpus

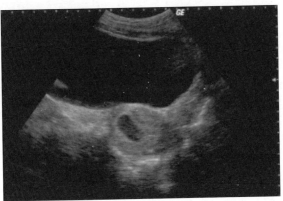

Fig. 2.5: In an overdistended urinary bladder the structures behind are going to get compressed and quite often the gestational sac shape gets distorted. In the picture see the urinary bladder well past the uterine fundus, causing discomfort to the patient. So best thing is to tell the patient to void and come back

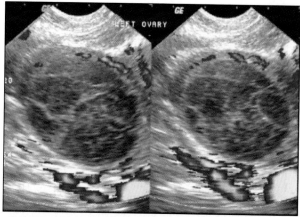

Fig. 2.6: Note that there are multiple areas within the lesion which are darker than the surrounding normal tissue. This is what is called as a hypoechoic lesion

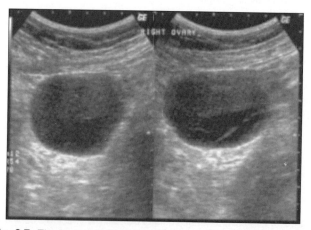

Fig. 2.7: The lesion which is completely black with distal acoustic enhancement is referred to as anechoic. Note that just adjacent to the lesion inferiorly is a bright white portion. This is what is distal acoustic enhancement

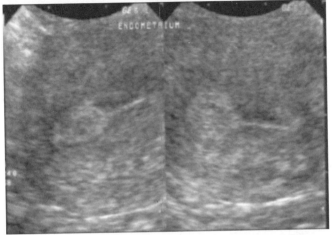

Fig. 2.8: Note that the lesion is brighter than the surrounding normal tissue. This is what is called as a hyperechoic lesion

gel. Additional gel should be placed on the outside of sheathed tip. The probe is inserted by a gentle push posteriorly towards the rectum while the patient relaxes. After removal of the transvaginal probe, the sheath is removed and the coupling gel is wiped off with a damp towel. It may be disinfected by Cidex. Three basic maneuvers are possible.

i. Advancement or withdrawal along the axis of the vagina.

ii. Angling by pointing the tip from side to side or anterior to posterior.

iii. Rotating the transducer along its axis.

10. Whatever you see on ultrasound is referred in terms of its echogenecity to adjacent organs as isoechoic, hypoechoic (Fig. 2.6), anechoic (Fig. 2.7) or hyperechoic (Fig. 2.8).

CHAPTER 3

Pregnancy with a Normal First Trimester (04-12 Weeks)

During an ultrasound examination you basically have these views.

1. With the transducer parallel to the midline scan from one side to the other looking at both the adnexa and the uterus.

2. With the transducer perpendicular to the midline scan from top to bottom looking at both the adnexa and the uterus (fundus to cervix).

3. Oblique sections to look at the fetus in detail. Depending on the position of the fetus try and get a longitudinal section of the fetus to measure crown rump length.

In order the structures one should be seeing in the first trimester are:

1. Uterus: This is where an intrauterine pregnancy is going to be seen. Be careful to evaluate the uterine cavity nicely especially in the fundus (Fig. 3.1), in the corpus (Fig. 3.2) and near the cornual areas.

2. Gestational sac: This is the anechoic area seen in the uterine cavity in cases of an intrauterine pregnancy (Fig. 3.3). Be

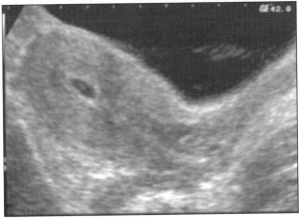

Fig. 3.1: The gestational sac is located in the uterine fundus

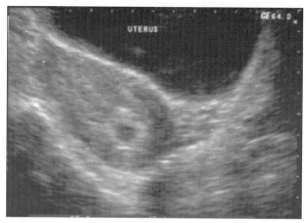

Fig. 3.2: The gestational sac is located in the uterine corpus

careful of not mistaking a pseudo-gestational sac for a gestational sac and the only way to differentiate is by seeing the yolk sac and embryo within it or seeing whether it is

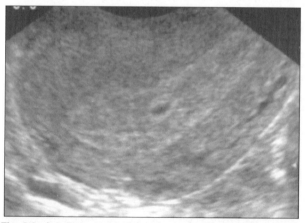

Fig. 3.3: Gestational sac: This is the anechoic area seen in the uterine cavity in cases of an intrauterine pregnancy

thick walled or not. When you start doing ultrasounds one starts recognizing gestational sacs at 5-5 1/2 weeks. Look for the number of gestational sacs (Fig. 3.4).

3. Yolk sac: Another circular anechoic area within the gestational sac (Fig. 3.5). This is the first sign which tells us that it is a healthy gestational sac.

4. Embryo: You start appreciating an embryo as early as 5 1/2 weeks (Fig. 3.6) with subtle cardiac activity which gets more and more clearer as gestational age advances. In the beginning you might be able to appreciate it around 6-6 1/2 weeks (Fig. 3.7). The heart rate is around 100 beats per minute in the beginning and increases to >130 beats per minute around 7 weeks (Fig. 3.8).

5. Trophoblastic reaction: The hyperechoic area around the gestational sac should be thick enough (02-04 mm) (Fig. 3.9) to ascertain whether the trophoblastic reaction is good or not.

6. Liquor amnii: The anechoic area inside the gestational sac excluding the embryo/fetus and yolk sac is the liquor amnii.

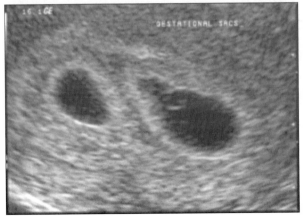

Fig. 3.4: Two separate gestational sacs seen in the uterine cavity

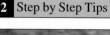

Fig. 3.5: Yolk sac: Another circular anechoic area within the gestational sac (arrow). This is the first sign which tells us that it is a healthy gestational sac

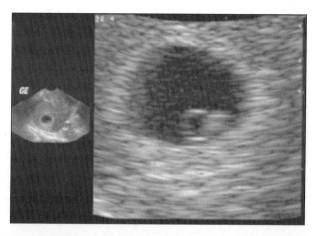

Fig. 3.6: Embryo: You start appreciating an embryo as early as 5 1/2 weeks as a small bleb adjacent to the yolk sac. If you concentrate one can see peristalsis/cardiac flicker within that small embryo

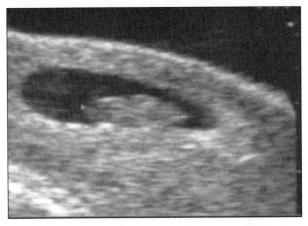

Fig. 3.7: One starts appreciating the embryo/fetus as it grows in size. An 8 weeks fetus with a circular portion and an ovoid portion

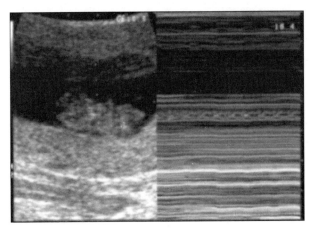

Fig. 3.8: The heart rate is around 100 beats per minute in the beginning and increases to >130 beats per minute around 7 weeks. An 08 weeks fetus with a good cardiac activity

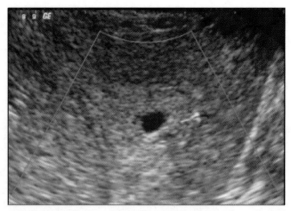

Fig. 3.9: Trophoblastic reaction: The hyperechoic area around the gestational sac should be thick enough (02-04 mm) to ascertain whether the trophoblastic reaction is good or not. Good thick trophoblastic reaction around a 51/2 weeks gestational sac

Assess the gestational sac size and embryo size to see whether it is adequate or not (Fig. 3.10).

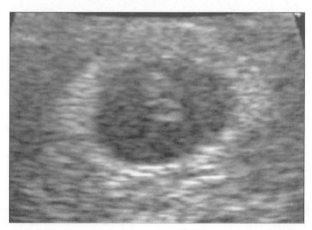

Fig. 3.10: Enough liquor amnii seen around the embryo and yolk sac

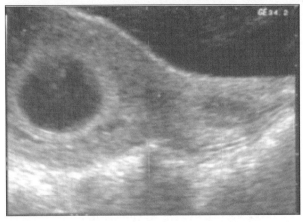

Fig. 3.11: Even in the first trimester always evaluate the cervical length by measuring from the cervical waist or the location of the internal os till the portion where the mucus plug ends. Any herniation or shortening to be reported for serial evaluation

7. Separation: Any anechoic area or hypoechoic area around the gestational sac denotes separation. Check the patient's history of any bleeding or spotting. Be very careful not to mistake unobliterated cavity for separation.
8. Cervix: Check the cervical length routinely on an adequately full bladder. Very full bladder elongates the cervix due to pressure. Look at the cervical canal and the mucus plug (hyperechoic) (Fig. 3.11).

On chapter 3 assess how fluent you are getting with the machine controls and try one or two cases of early normal (07-08 weeks) pregnancy. Try and assess the heartbeat and show it to your patient as well.

CHAPTER 4

Interaction with the Pregnancy and Fetus

1. Start looking inside the gestational sac in greater detail. Look very meticulously inside and differentiate the embryo from the yolk sac (Fig. 4.1) and measure them separately (Fig. 4.2). Change in size of the embryo by a mm can change the gestational age and the dating of the pregnancy is then erroneous.

2. You can see a thin curved line within the gestational sac, that is the amnion (Fig. 4.3).

3. As the pregnancy advances start differentiating the fetus into a head and a trunk portion after 08 weeks (Fig. 4.4).

4. Start measuring the embryo from one end to the other. Do not include the yolk sac. This measurement is called the crown rump length (CRL) (Fig. 4.5).

5. Start measuring the fetus from the top of the head to the bottom of the bottoms and do not include the limbs in this measurement (Fig. 4.6). This measurement is called the crown rump length (CRL).

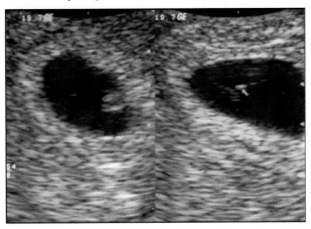

Fig. 4.1: The embryo is seen adjacent to the yolk sac. Be careful in differentiating between them. The yolk sac is the circular area within the gestational sac

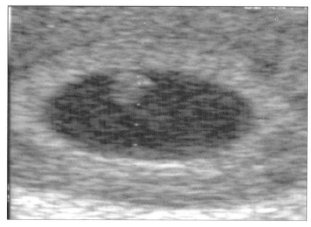

Fig. 4.2: Start looking inside the gestational sac in greater detail and measure the embryo and yolk sac separately. Change in size of the embryo by a mm can change the gestational age and the dating of the pregnancy is then erroneous

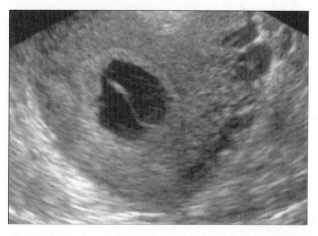

Fig. 4.3: The thin curved line within the gestational sac is the amnion

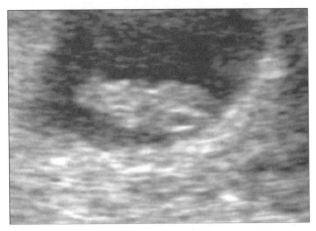

Fig. 4.4: The fetus can now be differentiated into a head and a trunk portion after 08 weeks

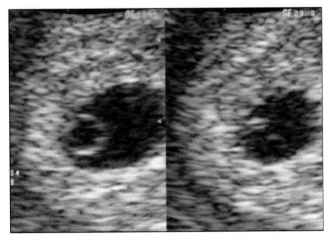

Fig. 4.5: The embryo measurement from one end to the other excluding the yolk sac is called the crown rump length (CRL)

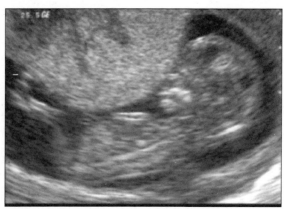

Fig. 4.6: The measurement of the fetus from the top of the head to the bottom of the bottoms excluding the limbs is called the crown rump length (CRL)

6. The crown rump length measurements with the gestational age come automatically on the screen/monitor (Fig. 4.7).

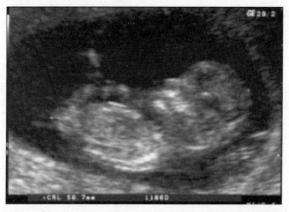

Fig. 4.7: The crown rump length measurements in mm/cm with the corresponding gestational age come automatically on the screen/monitor

7. Start looking for multiple sacs or multiple fetuses in the same sac.

8. If in very early pregnancy, upto 6 weeks if you are not sure about the cardiac activity please do not label as 'not present' but as "not seen as yet." Do not call it a missed abortion to find later that the pregnancy is carrying on. One can find embryonic bradycardia in a very early pregnancy (Fig. 4.8).

9. After 08 weeks one side of the gestational sac starts getting to be more thicker and hyperechoic. This is the area where the placental site is going to form (Fig. 4.9).

10. After 10 weeks one can see fetal anatomy also nicely. Try and appreciate the fetal cranium (Fig. 4.10) [choroid plexus (Fig. 4.11)], neck [nuchal translucency (Fig. 4.12)], face [orbits (Fig. 4.13) and nasal bone (Fig. 4.14)], spine

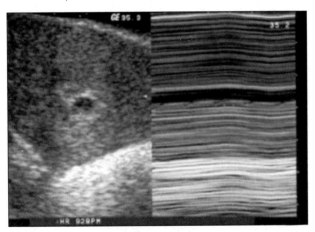

Fig. 4.8: Embryonic bradycardia in a very early pregnancy. Rather than giving a grim prognosis, it is always better to evaluate the patient again after 7-10 days and look for cardiac activity. One can see an embryonic heart rate of 92 beats per minute in a 5 weeks 4 days embryo

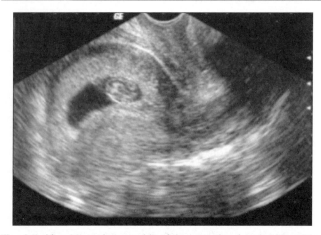

Fig. 4.9: After 08 weeks one side of the gestational sac starts getting to be more thicker and hyperechoic. This is the area where the placental site is going to form. Placental site seen on the anterior wall

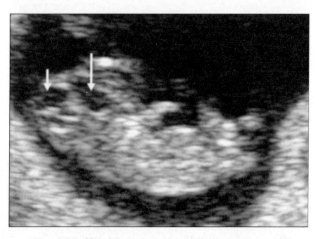

Fig. 4.10: After 08 weeks in the fetal cranium one can see these anechoic areas which are normal

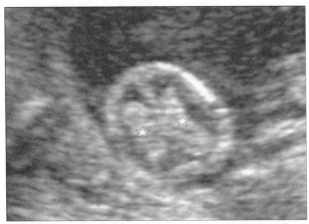

Fig. 4.11: Choroid plexuses (stars) seen in the fetal cranium. One can diagnose early gross hydrocephalus by viewing these choroid plexuses

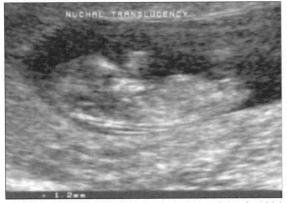

Fig. 4.12: Nuchal translucency in a 10 weeks 5 days fetus. Any thickening of the nuchal translucency prompts to a diagnosis of cystic hygroma, chromosomal abnormalities or cardiac abnormalities. Nuchal translucency thickness usually increases with gestational age with 1.5 mm and 2.5 mm being the 50th and 95th percentile respectively for gestational ages between 10 and 12 weeks. 2.0 mm and 3.0 mm are the 50th and 95th percentile respectively for gestational ages between 12 and 14 weeks

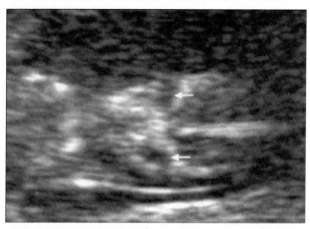

Fig. 4.13: Orbits (arrow) delineated as early as 11 weeks. Measure the ocular diameter, interocular distance and binocular distance to diagnose hypotelorism. Visualization of both orbits excludes anophthalmia or single orbit deformity

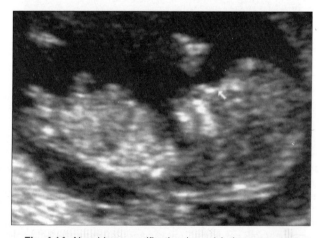

Fig. 4.14: Nasal bone ossification (arrow) being present or absent is a marker for Trisomy especially Trisomy 21

(Fig. 4.15), trunk [thoracic and abdominal viscera (Figs 4.16 to 4.18)] and limbs (Fig. 4.19). Be careful of not reporting herniation of bowel contents (omphalocele) in the first trimester as this is physiological (Fig. 4.20).

11. If the patient is bleeding look for any separation which looks like a hypoechoic area in any region around the gestational sac (Fig. 4.21).

12. Now start looking around for cervical length, any uterine masses, any adnexal masses and locate the site of corpus luteum.

13. The cervix is to be measured from the cervical waist till the lower limit by seeing the mucus plug which is seen as a hyperechoic area within the cervical canal.

14. Look at the uterine musculature (myometrium) for any masses (fibroids) (Fig. 4.22). Try and see the location (whether impinging on the uterine cavity or gestational sac or cervical canal) and measure the size for serial evaluation.

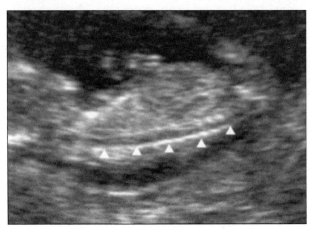

Fig. 4.15: Fetal spine can be seen as two parallel lines

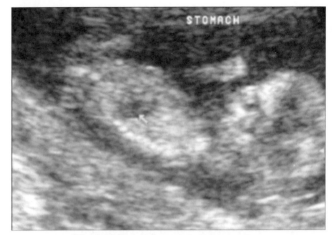

Fig. 4.16: Fetal stomach bubble seen in a fetus of 11 weeks and 4 days

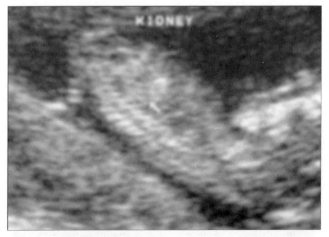

Fig. 4.17: Fetal kidney seen as an echogenic structure adjacent to the fetal spine

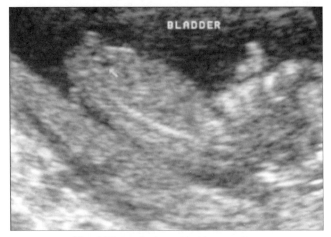

Fig. 4.18: Fetal urinary bladder seen in a fetus of 12 weeks and 2 days

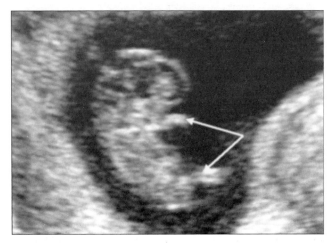

Fig. 4.19: Upper and lower limbs (arrow) seen

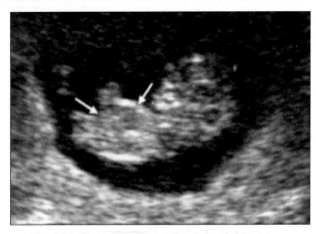

Fig. 4.20: Physiological herniation (arrow) of bowel seen below the umbilical cord

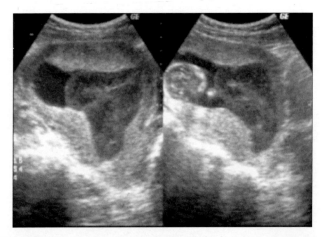

Fig. 4.21: The placenta is anterior with an amnio-decidual separation seen in the anterior wall superior to the cervix. This has an associated collection of 8.35 ml

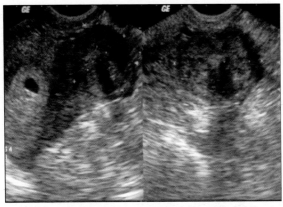

Fig. 4.22: Posterior wall fibroid which is panmural as it is impinging on the uterine cavity with a gestational sac in the uterine fundus

15. Look at both the adnexa (regions on the sides of the uterus) for any masses, which could commonly be ovarian or para-ovarian cysts, broad ligament fibroids or dermoids.

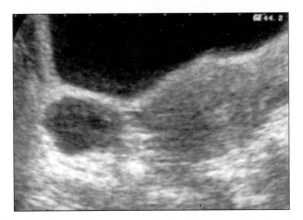

Fig. 4.23: Hypoechoic area seen in the right ovary with a 5 week and 6 days intrauterine pregnancy. This is the corpus luteum

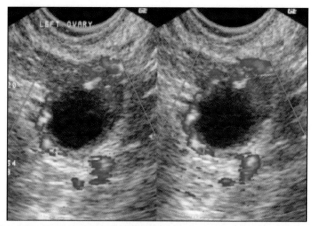

Fig. 4.24: If one has a color Doppler machine with the color flow map, one can visualize the corpus luteum vascularity so nicely

16. Look in for any anechoic or hypoechoic area (Figs 4.23 and 4.24) in the ovary on either side. This is the corpus luteum and is very helpful to diagnose from which side the follicle came from and to assess the tubal area nicely if no gestational sac is seen within the uterus.

CHAPTER 5

Abnormal Intrauterine Gestational Sac

1. Do not jump to the conclusion in the first instance that it is an abnormal pregnancy. There are specific criteria regarding an abnormal pregnancy.

2. Do not always depend on the patient's menstrual history. Go by last menstrual period date, regularity of periods and the date of the positive urine test for pregnancy to define how old the pregnancy possibly could be.

3. If you can see an embryo which is more than 05 mm in crown rump length and you do not see any cardiac pulsations it is an abnormal pregnancy (Fig. 5.1).

4. If the gestational sac is larger than 08 mm and you cannot delineate a yolk sac it is an abnormal pregnancy (Fig. 5.2).

5. If the gestational sac is larger than 16 mm and you cannot delineate an embryo it is an abnormal pregnancy (Fig. 5.3).

6. If you see an irregular amniotic sac, meaning the shape is not uniform (round or oval) with the criteria of no yolk sac or embryo it is an abnormal pregnancy (Figs 5.4 and 5.5).

7. Till 6 ½-7 weeks one can expect bradycardia. But if there is embryonic bradycardia (less than 120 beats per minute) even after that, there could be chances of this pregnancy not growing properly.

8. You have calculation on your machine to calculate the gestational age by gestational sac measurements and by crown rump length measurements. If you find that there is a considerable variation of more than 1-2 weeks this sac could be an oligo-amniotic sac (if gestational sac measurement is less than embryo measurement). Otherwise a quick way to diagnose is mean sac diameter minus crown rump length less than 5 mm. Oligo-amniotic sac one should be careful in the second trimester to look for any anomalies (Fig. 5.6).

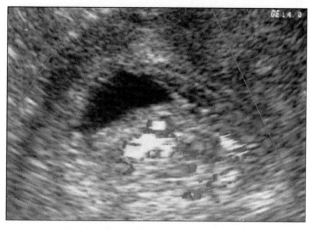

Fig. 5.1: No cardiac activity seen in this
08 mm pulseless attenuated embryo

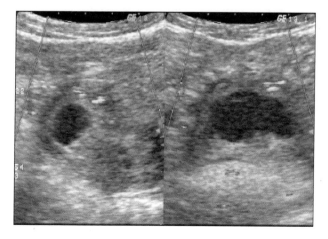

Fig. 5.2: Thin-walled gestational sac of 15 mm in the uterine
fundus with no embryo or yolk sac seen

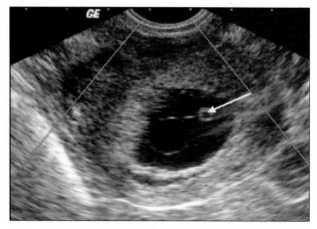

Fig. 5.3: Seven weeks gestational sac
showing a yolk sac but no embryo

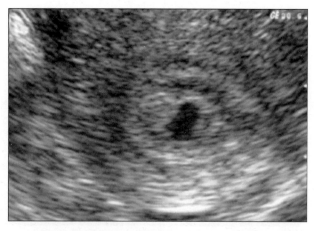

Fig. 5.4: Gestational sac of 6 weeks and 4 days
with a thin trophoblastic reaction. Note the gestational
sac shape is not round and regular

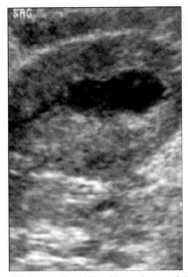

Fig. 5.5: Large, flaccid and irregular amniotic sac with a pulseless embryo

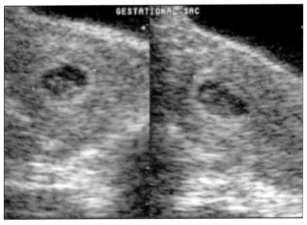

Fig. 5.6: Note that the sac is oligo-amniotic with the gestational sac corresponding less than the embryo size

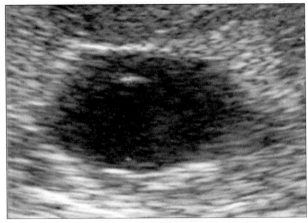

Fig. 5.7: Large yolk sac with the embryo seen adjacent to it

9. If the interval growth is poor again expect an impending pregnancy failure. This means that in a period of three weeks the gestational sac/embryo growth is much less than that.

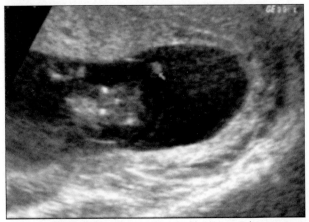

Fig. 5.8: Shrunken yolk sac with an extensive cystic hygroma associated with it

10. If the yolk sac is large (> 5.6 mm prior to 10 weeks) (Fig. 5.7)/small, shrunken or hyperechoic (Fig. 5.8) look out for fetal well being serially and in the second trimester for anomalies.

11. These are the points one should remember before giving a diagnosis of an abnormal intrauterine gestational sac.

12. If there is any doubt whatsoever revaluate the patient again after a week rather than giving a doubtful diagnosis.

CHAPTER 6

Abnormal Pregnancy: First Trimester

If the pregnant patient is bleeding and one has to detect the status, the points one should remember are:

1. Check whether you can see an intrauterine gestational sac (Fig. 6.1).
2. Check the cavity echoes as they are thin and usually homogeneous in cases of complete abortion (Fig. 6.2). If you have a color Doppler unit one can see a minimal uterine vascularity (warm or cold vascularity) (Fig. 6.3).
3. The cavity echoes are inhomogeneous and thickened in cases of incomplete abortion (Fig. 6.4). On a color Doppler unit one can see an overall diffuse increase in uterine vascularity (warm or hot vascularity) (Fig. 6.5).
4. The cavity is packed with echogenic tissue interspersed with numerous punctate sonolucencies in cases of molar change (Figs 6.6 and 6.7). On a color Doppler unit one can see an overall increase in uterine vascularity especially near areas of tumor invasion in the myometrium (Fig. 6.8).

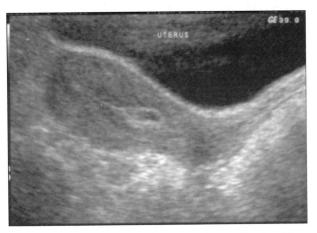

Fig. 6.1: Patient with bleeding per vaginum with a flaccid gestational sac in the uterine corpus

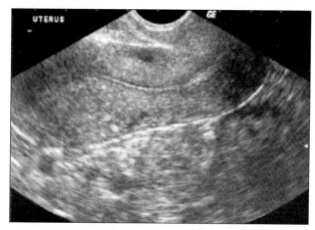

Fig. 6.2: A case of complete spontaneous abortion with very thin cavity echoes, 03-04 mm

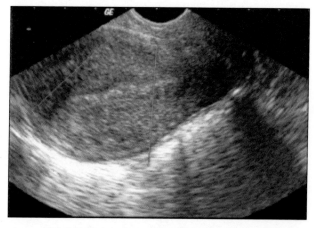

Fig. 6.3: The uterine vascularity is usually cold in a case of complete spontaneous abortion

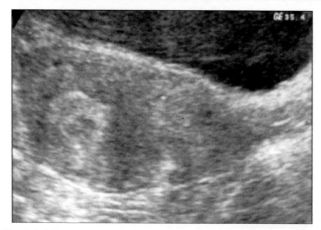

Fig. 6.4: Inhomogeneous echoes within the uterine cavity seen on 2D ultrasound in a case of amenorrhea 6 weeks with bleeding for 3 days

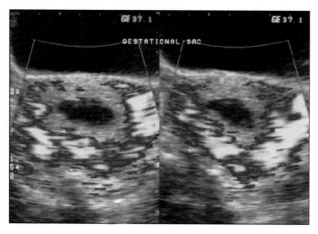

Fig. 6.5: Case of missed abortion seen on 2D ultrasound and on color Doppler, the overall uterine vascularity is increased (warm or hot vascularity)

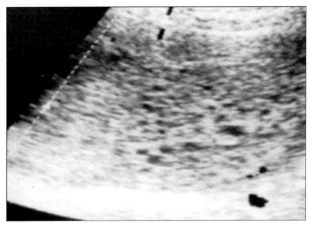

Fig. 6.6: Characteristic cystic spaces packed in the uterine cavity are seen in this case of molar pregnancy

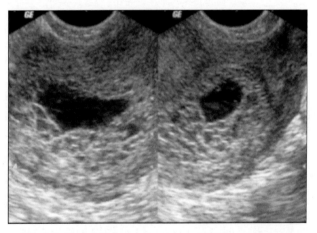

Fig. 6.7: Non-viable gestational sac with thin-walled clear cystic spaces around the gestational sac

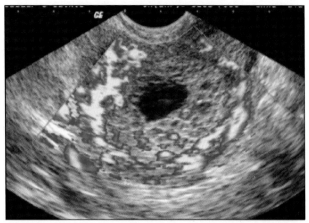

Fig. 6.8: In molar pregnancy in uncomplicated cases only mild increase in peri-lesional vascularity is noted. In invasive moles very high velocity flow in areas of tumor invasion within the myometrium are seen

5. If the urine test is positive and the patient is sure of the menstrual history and you do not see an intrauterine gestational sac one needs to diagnose ectopic pregnancy by these criteria.

   a. If you can see a gestational sac with a yolk sac and a pulsating embryo inside it in the adnexa, it is diagnostic of ectopic pregnancy (Fig. 6.9).

   b. If you do not see a gestational sac but the suspicion is very high look for other non-specific findings like an adnexal mass (Fig. 6.10), free fluid in the pouch of Douglas (Fig. 6.11), adnexa (Fig. 6.12) and sometimes even in the upper abdomen especially near the kidneys.

   c. The other non-specific findings on a color Doppler are a tubal vascular ring (Figs 6.13 and 6.14) and identification of adnexal peri-trophoblastic low-impedance flow.

   d. Corpus luteal flow is identified in one or both ovaries.

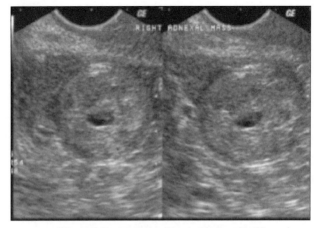

Fig. 6.9: Live ectopic with a gestational sac, yolk sac and an embryo with cardiac activity

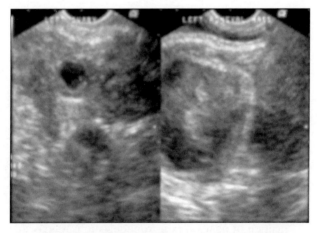

Fig. 6.10: Adnexal mass with corpus luteum in the left ovary with an adjacent inhomogeneous adnexal mass

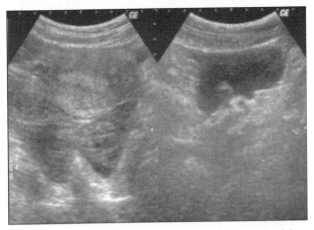

Fig. 6.11: Adnexal mass with free fluid (pelvic hematocele) in the pouch of Douglas and the left adnexa

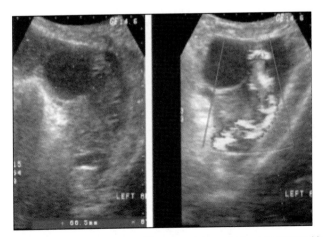

Fig. 6.12: Left adnexal mass with corpus luteum in the left ovary with an adjacent inhomogeneous adnexal mass and peri-lesional fluid collection

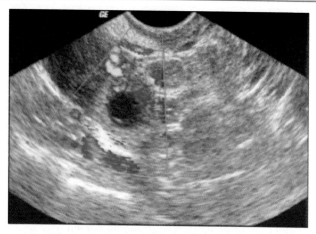

Fig. 6.13: On color Doppler in an ectopic pregnancy which is unruptured with viable trophoblasts avascular ring is delineated with the blood flow characteristically showing low-impedance, high-diastolic flow

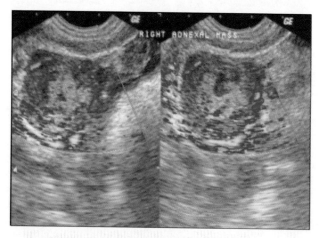

Fig. 6.14: Same case with marked peri-trophoblastic vascularity in the mass

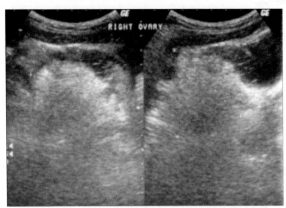

Fig. 6.15: Apart from the corpus luteum always evaluate the adnexa for any masses like dermoid, broad ligament fibroid or any other ovarian masses. Patient with an early pregnancy and an associated right ovarian dermoid

6. Make it a habit always to look at the adnexa irrespective of the intrauterine findings. You never know you could be looking at an ectopic or an ovarian mass (Fig. 6.15) or broad ligament fibroid.

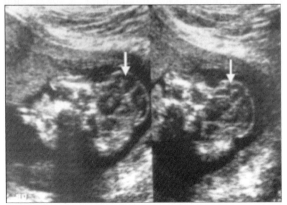

Fig. 6.16: Case of acrania with only brain and no bone seen superior to the orbits

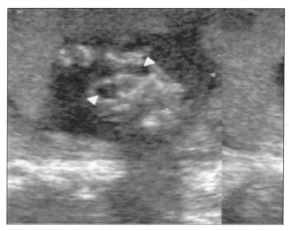

Fig. 6.17: Case of anencephaly with no brain or bone
seen superior to the orbits

7. In terms of anomalies, you should be able to delineate the
cranium and its gross abnormalities. Cranial anomalies like
acrania (Fig. 6.16) and anencephaly (Fig. 6.17). One should

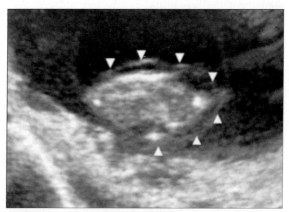

Fig. 6.18: Extensive cystic hygroma (arrow heads)
in a 10 weeks and 1 day fetus

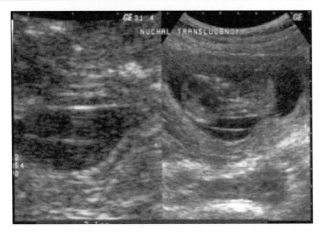

Fig. 6.19: Any thickening of the nuchal translucency prompts to a diagnosis of cystic hygroma, chromosomal abnormalities or cardiac abnormalities. Case of thickened nuchal translucency with abnormal biochemical markers in the first trimester

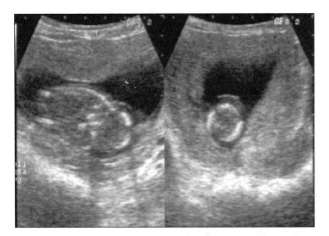

Fig. 6.20: Thickened nuchal translucency with persistent fetal bradycardia. Early amniocentesis revealed a chromosomal abnormality

be able to detect at 11 to 12 weeks. Fetal spine is seen as a double white line and any gross abnormality can be picked up. Extensive cystic hygroma can also be picked up at 10 to 11 weeks (Fig. 6.18).

8. Nuchal translucency thickness should be measured to assess for chromosomal abnormalities (Figs 6.19 and 6.20).

CHAPTER 7

First Trimester

FIRST TRIMESTER SCAN CHECK LIST

1. LMP and gestation
2. Identify uterus and gestational sac do not hesitate to do a transvaginal scan
3. Confirm viability and number
4. Look at the cervix and implantation site
5. Check adnexa
6. Measure embryo
7. Give a sonological gestational age and EDD and verify with LMP
8. Give a complete structured report with hard copy of pictures

FIRST TRIMESTER KEY POINTS

- CRL = 10 mm = mean for 7 weeks
- CRL = 30 mm = mean for 9 weeks 5 days
- CRL = 60 mm = mean for 12 weeks 3 days
- A viable intrauterine pregnancy practically rules out ectopic gestation (Except one in 30000)
- There is a delay of identifying of one week by trans-abdominal as compared to transvaginal

Sac (2-4 mm)	4.5 weeks	5.5 weeks
Fetal heart (CRL 2-4)	5 weeks	6 weeks
Yolk sac (10 mm)	5 weeks	6 weeks

- Early fetal bradycardia signifies poor prognosis
- Fetal chromosomal anomalies can be screened for and detected in the 10-14 weeks scan
- Transvaginal scan does not increase abortion risk of bleeding

- A thorough knowledge of fetal embryology and implantation and corpus luteum physiology is a must for first trimester diagnosis
- Do not hesitate to take second opinion
- 20 mm sac with no intra sac structures is suggestive of anembryonic pregnancy. A CRL of > 6 mm without fetal heart is suggestive of missed abortion. Confirm by TVS and repeat scan if required.

TRANSVAGINAL DECISION FLOW CHART

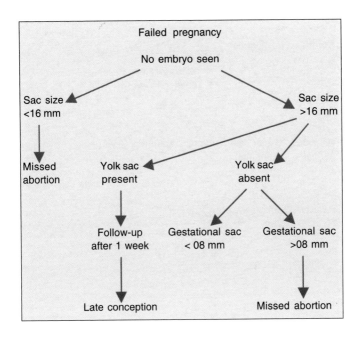

DECISION MAKING IN THE FIRST TRIMESTER

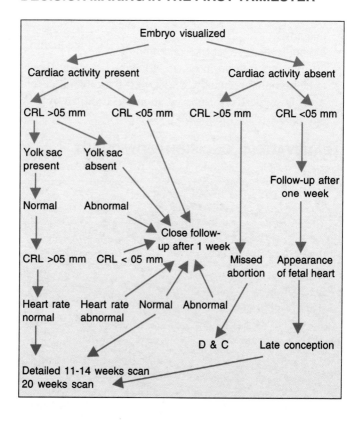

CHAPTER 8

Normal Second Trimester: Extra-Fetal

In the second trimester apart from the fetus you need to see around the fetus. The points one should be seeing are:

1. Placenta

   a. Location: Check the distance of the inferior limit of the placenta from the internal os (Fig. 8.1), so that next time you have an objective evaluation rather than a subjective one. If the distance is more than 30 mm it is usually regarded as normal. Apart from the distance check whether the placenta is on the anterior (Fig. 8.2), posterior (Fig. 8.3), right (Fig. 8.4) or left wall or is it fundal.

   b. Thickness: Refer to charts for week wise increase in thickness of the placenta. The variations are mentioned in the requisite day (Fig. 8.5).

   c. Focal lesion: The focal lesion, one should be most concerned about, is Chorioangioma as it has arterio-venous shunting and can cause congestive cardiac

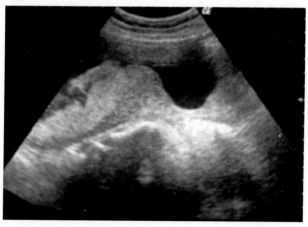

Fig. 8.1: The placenta in this case is far away from the internal os, so it is an upper segment placenta

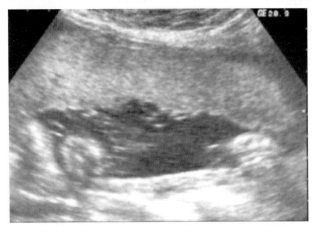

Fig. 8.2: As the placenta is on the wall closer to the transducer it is an anterior placenta

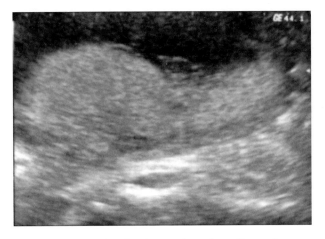

Fig. 8.3: Note that the placenta is on the wall away from the transducer, therefore it is a posterior placenta

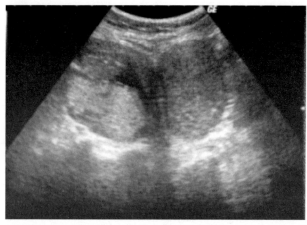

Fig. 8.4: On a transverse section the placenta is seen on the left of the screen, therefore it is a right wall placenta and it is *vice versa* for a left wall placenta

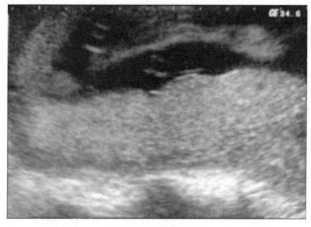

Fig. 8.5: The thickness of the placenta varies with increasing gestational age. So refer to the charts for the measurements

status. The other focal lesions usually do not cause a decrease in placental reserve (Fig. 8.6).

   d. Echo pattern: There are various grades of placenta like Grade 0 (Fig. 8.7), I (Fig. 8.8), II and III.

   e. Retroplacental area: Usually appears hypoechoic because of vessels, so do not mistake it as retroplacental collection (Fig. 8.9).

2. Liquor Amnii

   a. Calculate the amniotic fluid index to see whether the liquor amnii is normal in quantity or not (Fig. 8.10).

   b. Fetal swallowing and urinary flow are the primary regulators of amniotic fluid. So abnormalities of these systems cause oligohydramnios (decreased liquor amnii) or polyhydramnios (increased liquor amnii) which can be indirect signs for detecting anomalies.

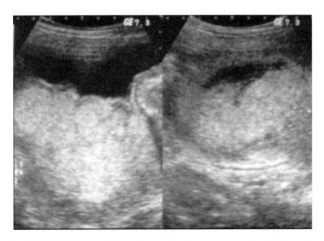

Fig. 8.6: Multiple anechoic or hypoechoic areas near the fetal surface or the uterine surface of the placenta are seen. The only focal lesion of significance is chorioangioma which is hypoechoic and very vascular

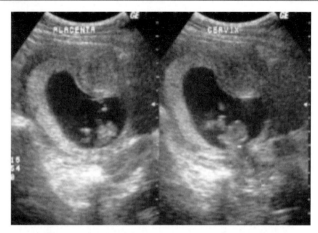

Fig. 8.7: Grade 0 placenta at 13 weeks and 6 days

3. Umbilical Cord
   a. Check for number of vessels as there should be two
      arteries and one vein in the umbilical cord.

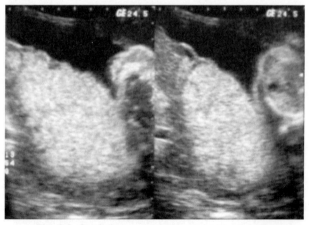

Fig. 8.8: Grade I placenta at 20 weeks and 2 days

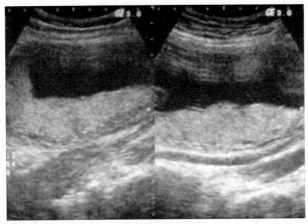

Fig. 8.9: The retroplacental area usually appears hypoechoic because of vessels, so do not mistake it as retroplacental collection

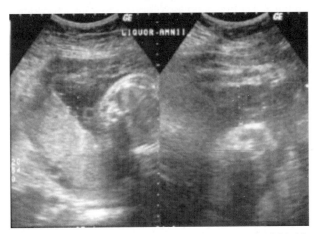

Fig. 8.10: Amniotic fluid index assessment. The uterus is divided into four quadrants by the midline and transverse axis and the amniotic fluid as the deepest vertical pocket free of fetal parts and umbilical cord is measured in each quadrant and all four quadrants add up to give the amniotic fluid index

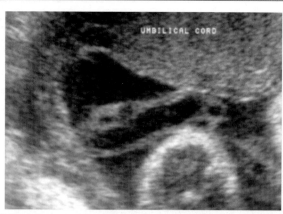

Fig. 8.11: Three vessel cord as seen on 2D ultrasound. The single umbilical vein and two umbilical arteries are seen as a rail track appearance

    b. In a 2D ultrasound look for the rail track appearance to assess for number of vessels (Figs 8.11 to 8.13).

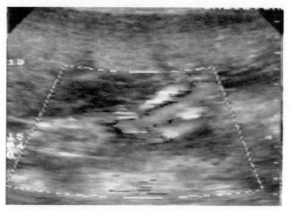

Fig. 8.12: Three vessel cord as seen on color flow mapping. Two umbilical arteries (blue) and single umbilical vein (red) can be easily demonstrated. On color flow mapping the red and blue to not specify arteries and veins but flow towards the transducer or away from it

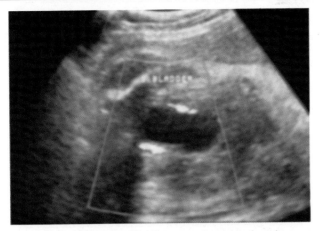

Fig. 8.13: Hypogastric arteries seen adjacent to the urinary bladder on both sides confirming a three vessel cord

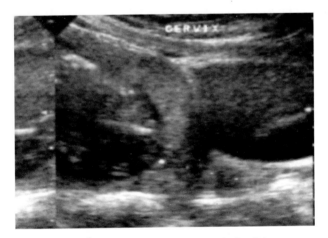

Fig. 8.14: The internal os should be seen whether it is open or not and whether there is any herniation as well

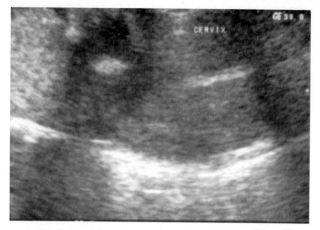

Fig. 8.15: Length: The cervical length is measured from the internal os to the external os or the mucus plug is measured

4. Cervix
   a. Internal os: Look for internal os, open or not (Fig. 8.14) and whether there is any herniation as well. Upto 05 mm without herniation is normal, 05 to 08 mm is borderline and more than 08 mm one labels it as cervical incompetence. Irrespective of the dimensions of the internal os if there is any herniation of the amnion it is an incompetent cervix.
   b. Length: The cervical length is measured from the internal os to the external os (Fig. 8.15). More than 30 mm is normal, 25 to 30 mm is borderline and less than 25 mm is a short cervix.
5. Myometrium and Adnexa
   a. Masses: Look for any fibroids or any ovarian or extra-ovarian adnexal masses.

CHAPTER 9

Normal Second Trimester: Fetal Evaluation

Apart from checking the number of fetuses and their viability the fetus should be evaluated for normalcy and age. The basic points of scanning the fetus are:

1. Look at the cranium for presence of brain and bone.
2. Evaluate the cranium in the three basic sections:
   a. Section for cranial biometry in which you see the thalamus pointing posteriorly and the cavum septum pellucidum anteriorly (Fig. 9.1).
   b. Parallel to this section superiorly is the section for the lateral ventricles (Fig. 9.2).
   c. Come back to the section for cranial biometry and rotate the transducer in such a way that the center being constant the posterior portion of the transducer angles inferiorly around 30 to 45 degrees till you see the posterior cranial fossa structures *viz.* cerebellum (Fig. 9.3) and cisterna magna (Fig. 9.4).

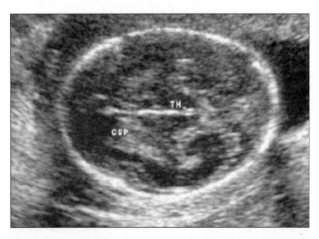

Fig. 9.1: Section for cranial biometry. The thalamus should be in the center and cavum septum pellucidum anteriorly with the cerebellum and cisterna magna not seen in the section

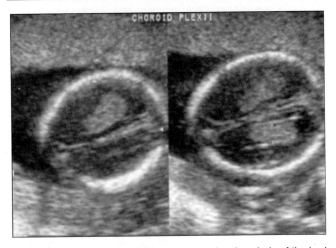

Fig. 9.2: Choroid plexuses (CP) seen occupying the whole of the body of the lateral ventricle. The anterior horn of the lateral ventricle and posterior horn of the lateral ventricle are not filled by the choroid plexuses. The width of the body of the lateral ventricle, the inter-hemispheric distance and the ratio of the width of the body of the lateral ventricle to the inter-hemispheric distance is calculated. (Normal value < 50%). This is not sensitive for early hydrocephalus. The width of the body, anterior horn and posterior horn of the lateral ventricle are taken. (Normal value < 08 mm, Borderline 08-10 mm and > 10 mm abnormal)

3. Check the fetal neck for any masses.
4. Check the fetal spine for any breech in the cutaneous or subcutaneous elements or any disorganization of the osseous elements (Fig. 9.5).
5. Check the fetal face for any deformity of orbits or any dropout of upper lip echoes (Fig. 9.6).
6. Check the fetal thorax and see the heart, lungs and diaphragm (Fig. 9.7).
7. Check the fetal heart for situs, size, rate, rhythm, configuration and connections (Fig. 9.8).

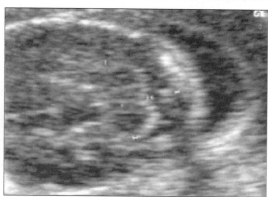

Fig. 9.3: The cerebellum is seen as a 'W' turned 90 degrees. The cerebellar hemispheres and the cerebellar vermis should be appreciated for posterior cranial fossa abnormalities. The cerebellar transverse diameter (CTD) is measured from the edges of both cerebellar hemispheres. The CTD in mm from 14-22 weeks is equal to the gestational age of the fetus in weeks

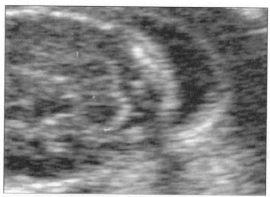

Fig. 9.4: The cisterna magna is seen posterior to the cerebellar vermis and anterior to the occipital bone. (Normal value < 08 mm, Borderline 08-10 mm and > 10 mm abnormal). Few strands seen traversing the cisterna magna are normal. Carefully check for any communication between the fourth ventricle and the cisterna magna with an abnormal cerebellar vermis. If there is any communication at gestational age less than 16 weeks revaluate the fetus after 2 weeks

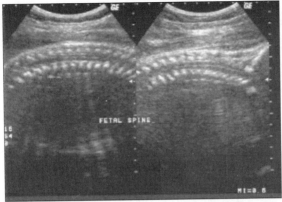

Fig. 9.5: The longitudinal plane delineates the soft tissue components posterior to the spine and dysraphic disorganization of the spine. The cutaneous, subcutaneous and muscular components seen posterior to the vertebral column need to be carefully screened all along the cervical, dorsal, lumbar and sacrococcygeal vertebrae

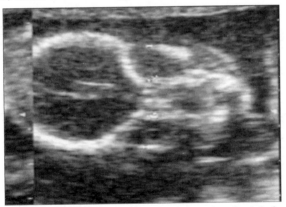

Fig. 9.6: Fetal orbits seen in the facial skeleton view. Look in for any contour abnormality and for any orbital calcification. The ocular diameter (both sides measurement of the orbit), interocular distance (measurement between the two eye sockets) and binocular distance (measurement from one eye socket to the other) to be measured to look for any hypo/hypertelorism which could be a stigmata specific for various syndromes

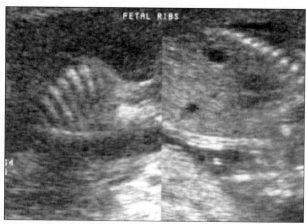

Fig. 9.7: In the fetal thorax look for any deformity of the ribs like crowding or narrowing. The diaphragm separates the thorax and abdomen and the heart and lungs to be seen superior to it and the stomach and liver to be seen inferior to it. Fetal lungs are seen for their echo pattern and to look for any masses

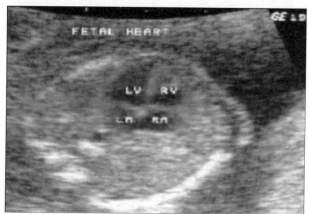

Fig. 9.8: Cardiac situs is seen in comparison with the fetal stomach being on the same side. Cardiac configuration is checked by visualizing all four chambers. (LV: left ventricle, LA: left atrium, RV: right ventricle and RA: right atrium)

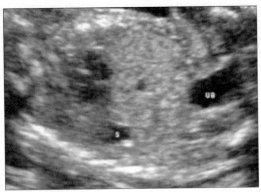

Fig. 9.9: Fetal stomach bubble to be seen. Revaluate again if stomach bubble not seen. See for a double bubble sign for duodenal atresia. Check small and large bowel echoes for any change in echo pattern or hyperperistalsis.Check the omentum and mesentery for any fluid collections or calcification

8. Check the fetal abdomen for stomach bubble (Fig. 9.9), kidneys (Fig. 9.10) and urinary bladder (Fig. 9.11).

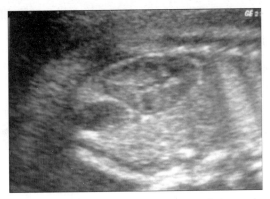

Fig. 9.10: Check fetal kidneys for abnormalities of situs, axis, contour, echo pattern and size. Fetal kidneys as seen in the third trimester with a mildly hypoechoic cortex and prominent pyramids

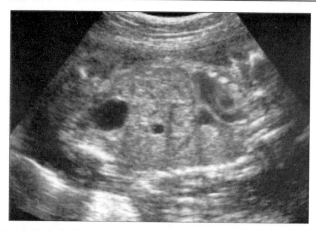

Fig. 9.11: Check for fetal kidneys and bladder contour and capacity. If you do not see the fetal bladder revaluate again. Look for any dilatation of the proximal urethra

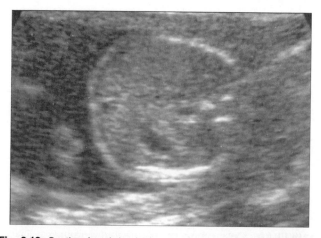

Fig. 9.12: Section for abdominal perimeter measurement. The spine should be posterior and the umbilical part of the portal vein anteriorly

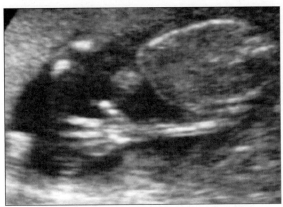

Fig. 9.13: Fetal hand. Visualize the fetal digits for any polydactyly or syndactyly

9. Measure the abdominal perimeter. For the section for abdominal perimeter measurement the spine should be posterior and the umbilical part of the portal vein anterior (Fig. 9.12).

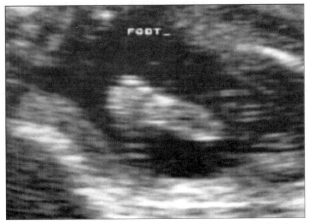

Fig. 9.14: Fetal foot. Apart from seeing the fetal limbs fetal feet to be seen for any club foot deformities

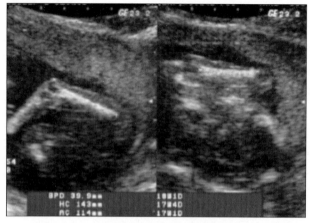

Fig. 9.15: Femoral and humeral length measurement
for any abnormalities of bone lengths

10. View the limbs and look for thigh, knee, leg, foot (Fig.
9.13), arm, fore-arm and hand (Fig. 9.14) on both sides.
Measure the femoral length in a complete longitudinal
section (Fig. 9.15).

CHAPTER 10

Extra-Fetal Variations: Second Trimester

1. Placenta
   a. Location: The placenta could be reaching upto the internal os or spanning across it (Fig. 10.1).
   b. Thickness: Usually a thickened placenta is seen in cases of maternal increase in Blood Sugar or in cases of Triploidy (Fig. 10.2). A thinned or shrunken placenta is seen in cases of Maternal infection or in cases of severe increase in Maternal Blood Pressure.
   c. Focal Lesion: There are multiple focal lesions spanning across the whole placenta on both surfaces. One is most concerned about Chorioangioma which appears as a hypoechoic extremely vascular lesion.
   d. Retroplacental Area: Depending on the stage of collection the appearance can be hypoechoic or sometimes even isoechoic to the placenta. One can also see a collection in the subchoriol area (fetal surface of the placenta) (Fig. 10.3).

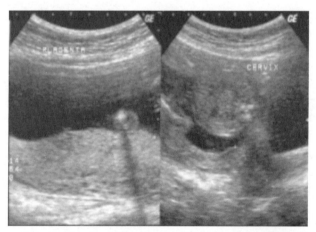

Fig. 10.1: The placenta is posterior. Its inferior limit extends down to the internal os but does not span across it

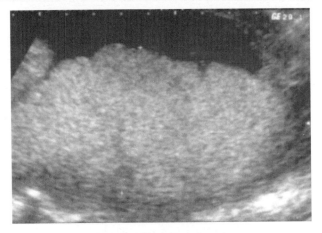

Fig. 10.2: Thickened placenta
(55 mm at 20 weeks and 2 days)

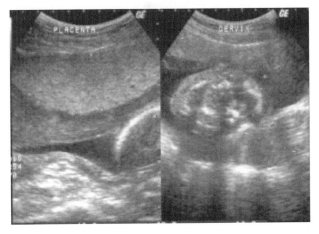

Fig. 10.3: Subchoriol collection. The placenta,
retroplacental area and fetus were normal

2. Liquor Amnii
    a. When liquor amnii is reduced it is called oligohydramnios (Fig. 10.4). Try and assess the reasons for oligohydramnios as it can be due to:
        i. Decreased urine production because of bilateral renal disease.
        ii. Post-compensatory sequelae of Intrauterine growth retardation.
        iii. Rupture of membranes.
    b. When liquor amnii is increased it is called polyhydramnios (Fig. 10.5). Try and assess the reasons for polyhydramnios as it can be due to:
        i. Open neural tube defects, e.g. Encephalocele, Meningomyelocele, Anencephaly.
        ii. Abnormalities primarily due to gastrointestinal obstruction, e.g. Esophageal atresia, duodenal

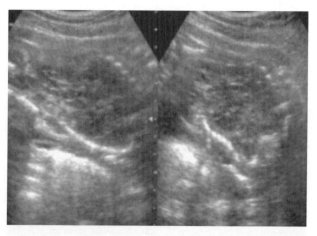

Fig. 10.4: Severe oligohydramnios in a case of bilateral renal agenesis. Note the complete absence of liquor amnii with the uterine wall closely opposed to the fetus

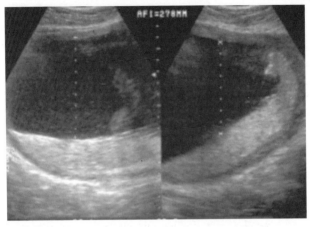

Fig. 10.5: Moderate polyhydramnios in a case of congenital diaphragmatic hernia. Diagnosis is striking in these cases as the fetus is seen freely mobile in liquor amnii. Both pockets shown in the picture are more than 80 mm each

atresia, small bowel atresia/obstruction or secondarily due to compression of the gastrointestinal system, e.g. Cystic adenomatoid malformation, mass in the mediastinum, diaphragmatic hernia commonly left side.

iii. Maternal diabetes mellitus.

iv. Fetal hydrops (immune or non-immune).

v. Chromosomal abnormality : Trisomy 18.

c. Amniotic bands : Whenever one sees amniotic bands in the uterine cavity traversing the gestational sac be careful of evaluating whether any fetal part is impinged upon by these bands causing limb reduction defects or any other external anomaly of the cranium, face, anterior abdominal wall or spine (Fig. 10.6).

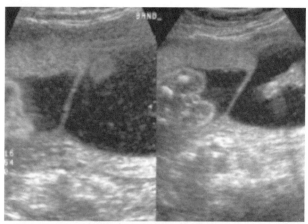

Fig. 10.6: Amniotic fold/band seen traversing the uterine cavity. Be careful to check for any limb or digit reduction/constriction defects, external anomalies of the face (cleft lip and palate, nasal abnormalities), cranum (anencephaly or encephalocele), anterior abdominal wall defects and abnormal curvature of the spine

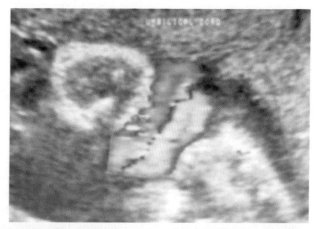

Fig. 10.7: Two vessel cord as seen on color flow mapping. Single umbilical artery (red) and single umbilical vein (blue) can be seen

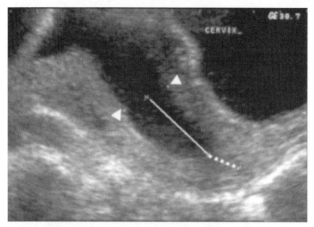

Fig. 10.8: Patient of cervical incompetence. The internal os (arrow heads) is open and 18 mm wide. The herniation of the amnion in the cervical canal (line) is over a distance of 32 mm. The functional or closed cervix (dashed line) which is required for the cerclage is 13 mm long

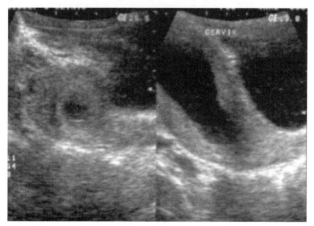

Fig. 10.9: Another patient of cervical incompetence with the cervix seen in a transverse section (right side) and longitudinal section (left side)

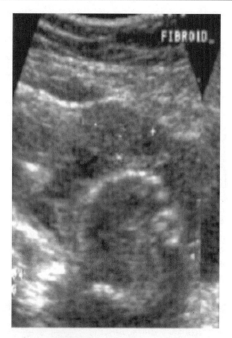

Fig. 10.10: An anterior wall subserous
fibroid in a 16 weeks pregnancy

3. Umbilical Cord
    a. Whenever a single umbilical artery (Fig. 10.7) is
       diagnosed a careful search for anomalies should be done
       especially chromosomal abnormalities, major cardiac
       defects, holoprosencephaly, anterior abdominal wall
       defects and skeletal deformities. With no other anomaly
       detected continuation of pregnancy can be thought of.
4. Cervix
    a. Internal os

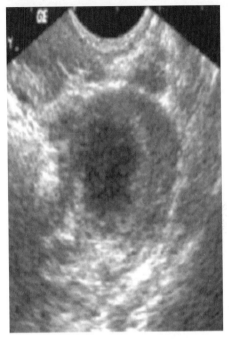

Fig. 10.11: Persistent corpus luteum
in a 19 weeks pregnancy

   b. Length Herniation of the amnion through an open
     internal os (Figs 10.8 and 10.9) or a short cervix
     are abnormalities in the cervix commonly
     encountered.
5. Myometrium and Adnexa
   a. Masses (Figs 10.10 and 10.11)

CHAPTER 11

Abnormal Second Trimester: Fetal Evaluation

1. If you do not see bone but only brain floating this is **Acrania** (Fig. 11.1).
2. If you do not see bone or brain above the orbits this is **Anencephaly** (Fig. 11.2).
3. If you a break in the osseous continuity of the cranium this is a **Meningocele/Encephalocele** (Figs 11.3 and 11.4).
4. If you see an anechoic circular area/areas in the choroid plexii these are **Choroid plexus cyst/s** (Fig. 11.5).
5. If you dilatation of the lateral ventricles with a dangling choroid plexus this is **Hydrocephalus** (Figs 11.3 to 11.9).
6. If you see an anechoic cavity in the brain commonly it is due to **Holoprosencephaly** (Fig. 11.10) or **Agenesis of the Corpus callosum** (Fig. 11.11).
7. If you see an increase in depth of the cisterna magna with cerebellar vermis hypoplasia and fourth ventricle

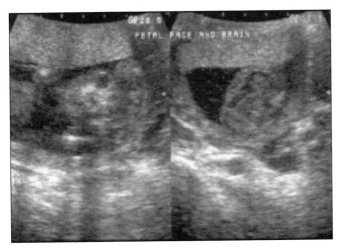

Fig. 11.1: Fetal acrania. Note the brain tissue but no osseous covering over it

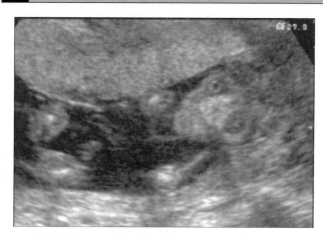

Fig. 11.2: Orbits seen with nothing seen superior to it (neither brain nor bone)

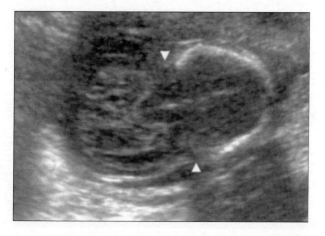

Fig. 11.3: Note the defect in the occipital bone (arrow heads) with the herniation of brain tissue from the defect

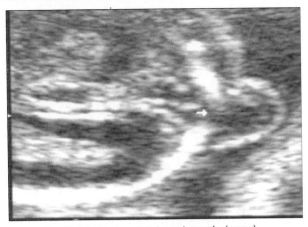

Fig. 11.4: Lateral occipital meningocele (arrow).
Note the clear contents within the herniated sac

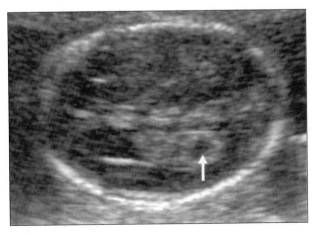

Fig. 11.5: Unilateral single (arrow) choroid plexus cyst. A detailed scan
to check for sonographic stigmata of chromosomal abnormalities
especially Trisomy 18 is done and only if any additional anomaly is
detected an amniocentesis is indicated for

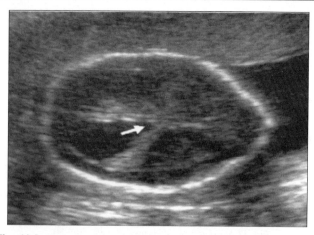

Fig. 11.6: Enlarged lateral ventricles with loss of the approximation between the choroid plexus and the medial border of the lateral ventricle. Choroid plexus occupies the whole of the body of the lateral ventricle. The width of the body of the lateral ventricle, the inter-hemispheric distance and the ratio of the width of the body of the lateral ventricle to the inter-hemispheric distance is calculated. (Normal value < 50%). This is not sensitive for early hydrocephalus. The width of the body, anterior horn and posterior horn of the lateral ventricle are taken. (Normal value < 08 mm, Borderline 08-10 mm and > 10 mm abnormal). When the choroid plexus does not occupy the whole of the body of the lateral ventricle see for the measurement of the medial separation (arrow) of the choroid plexus from the wall of the lateral ventricle. (Normal value < 02 mm, Borderline 02-03 mm and > 03 mm is abnormal)

communicating with the cisterna magna it is **Dandy-Walker malformation** (Fig. 11.12).

8. See the fetal neck for any thickening of the nuchal skin fold (Fig. 11.13).

9. If you see a septated mass posterior to the fetal neck this is a **Cystic hygroma** (Fig. 11.14).

10. If you see a break in the continuity of the cutaneous or subcutaneous or osseous components in the cervical,

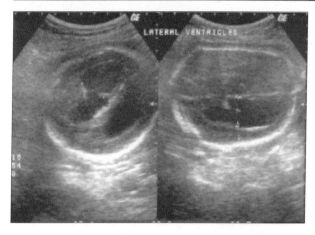

Fig. 11.7: Dangling choroid plexuses seen
in enlarged lateral ventricles

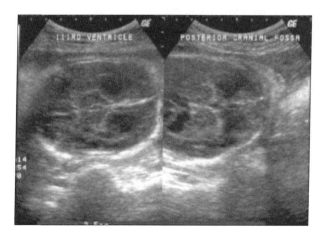

Fig. 11.8: Enlarged third ventricle with posterior cranial fossa
structures not adequately delineated because of herniation

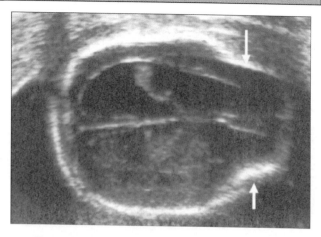

Fig. 11.9: Overlapping of the frontal bones (arrow) seen in a case of communicating hydrocephalus

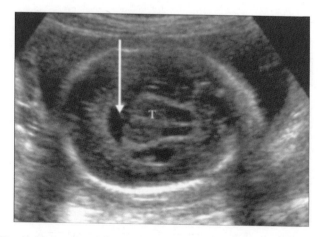

Fig. 11.10: Alobar holoprosencephaly with a dorsal sac (arrow) and a monoventricular cavity with a displaced cerebral cortex

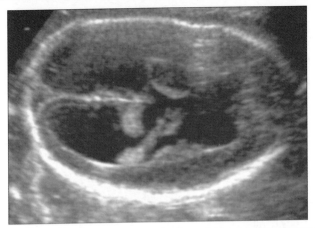

Fig. 11.11: Ventriculomegaly seen in the atrial and occipital regions (colpocephaly) because of poorly developed white matter surrounding these areas (Tear drop configuration) with an absent cavum septum pellucidum

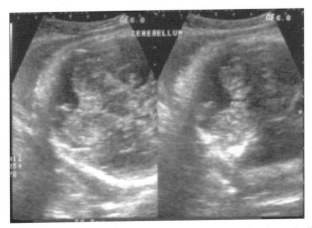

Fig. 11.12: Large cyst in the posterior cranial fossa with a hypoplastic cerebellar vermis. Midline cyst in the posterior cranial fossa which is communicating with the fourth ventricle

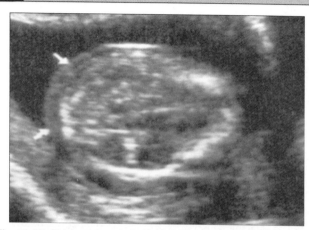

Fig. 11.13: Thickened nuchal skin fold with an associated ventricular septal defect. Amniocentesis revealed a Trisomy 21 karyotype. Nuchal skin fold thickness assessment through the section just inferior to the section for cerebellum and cisterna magna. (14-18 weeks : Normal value < 04 mm, Borderline 04-05 mm and > 05 mm requires further karyotypic analysis) (18-22 weeks : Normal value < 05 mm, Borderline 05-06 mm and > 06 mm requires further karyotypic analysis)

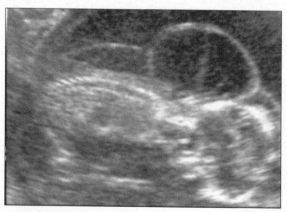

Fig. 11.14: Cystic hygroma (septated) seen in the longitudinal section posterior to the cranium, craniovertebral junction and cervical vertebra

dorsal, lumbar, sacral or coccygeal spine this is a **Spinal meningocele/meningomyelocele** (Figs 11.15 to 11.18).

11. Try and assess the fetal facial symmetry and the continuity of the upper lip. If there is a dropout of echoes this is a **Cleft lip**.

12. If you see an anechoic fluid collection in the fetal chest around the fetal lungs this is a **Pleural effusion** (Fig. 11.19).

13. If you see a cystic mass or a hyperechoic mass in the fetal lung this is a **Cystic adenomatoid malformation** (Fig. 11.20).

14. If you do not see the fetal stomach in the abdomen but in the thorax this is a **Congenital diaphragmatic hernia.**

15. If you see polyhydramnios and do not see a stomach bubble this is an **Esophageal atresia** (Fig. 11.21).

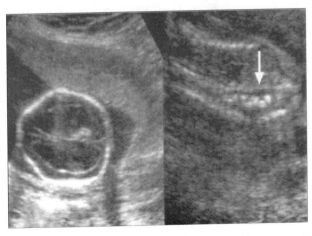

Fig. 11.15: Ventriculomegaly (left side) seen with a dysraphic disorganization of the lumbar and sacrococcygeal vertebrae (arrow)

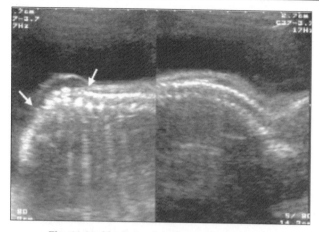

Fig. 11.16: Meningocele with anechoic contents

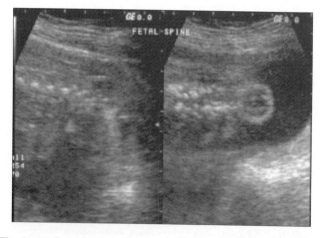

Fig. 11.17: Defect in the osseous component of the vertebral column and disruption of cutaneous and subcutaneous elements with a tethered spinal cord

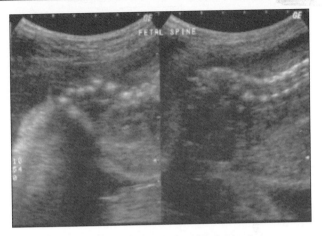

Fig. 11.18: Kyphoscoliosis of the fetal spine

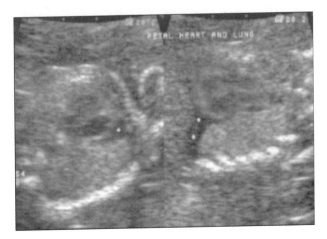

Fig. 11.19: Unilateral pleural effusion taking the shape of the chest wall and mediastinum

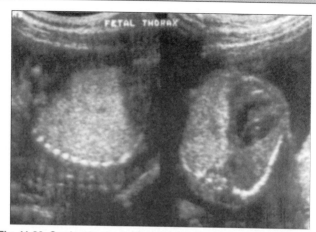

Fig. 11.20: Cystic adenomatoid malformation of the right lung. Because of distal acoustic enhancement from very small cysts the lesion appears as a solid mass. Note the difference in echo pattern from the left lung

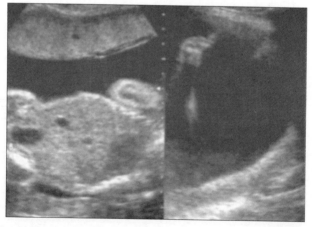

Fig. 11.21: Esophageal atresia as diagnosed by demonstration of polyhydramnios (right side) with an inability to visualize the stomach bubble (left side)

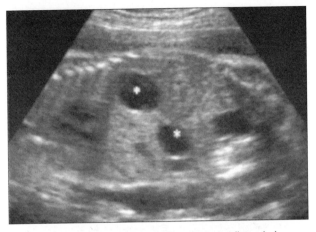

Fig. 11.22: Double bubble sign seen as a distended stomach and an enlarged duodenal bulb

16. If you see polyhydramnios and two bubbles in the fetal abdomen this is a **Duodenal atresia** (Fig. 11.22).

17. If you see an anechoic fluid collection in the fetal abdomen around the abdominal viscera this is **Ascites** (Fig. 11.23).

18. If you see dilatation of the renal calyces and pelvis this is **Hydronephrosis** (Fig. 11.24) and if accompanying it if you see a dilated ureter this is **Hydroureteronephrosis**.

19. If you see multiple thin walled clear cystic areas with a hyperechoic cortex in the fetal kidneys with or without oligohydramnios this is **Multicystic dysplastic kidney/s** (Fig. 11.25).

20. If you see multiple thin walled clear cystic areas in the fetal kidneys with oligohydramnios this is **Polycystic kidneys** (Fig. 11.26).

21. If on looking at the sole of the foot you can see the tibia this is a **Clubfoot deformity** (Fig. 11.27).

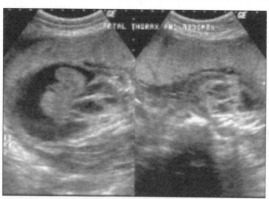

Fig. 11.23: Fetal ascites seen surrounding the fetal viscera

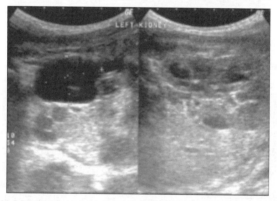

Fig. 11.24: Whenever you are reporting hydronephrosis, specify the dilated renal pelvis, dilated renal calyces, cortical thickness and echo pattern. Anteroposterior diameter of the renal pelvis. The values for the anteroposterior diameter of the renal pelvis (measured on a transverse view through the kidney) are from 15-20 weeks of gestation < 04 mm is normal, 04-07 mm is borderline and > 08 mm is abnormal or hydronephrotic. From 20 weeks onwards < 06 mm is normal, 06-09 is borderline and > 10mm is abnormal or hydronephrotic. Be careful that borderline cases are to be reviewed by serial scans before labeling them as hydronephrotic

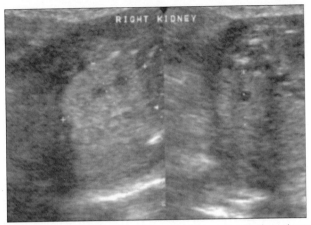

Fig. 11.25: Bilateral echogenic kidneys which are dysplastic and small with very less pelviectasis. This is not a reduction in hydronephrosis as the improvement with dysplastic kidney is because the renal function is poor or absent and is not going to improve even after the obstruction is corrected

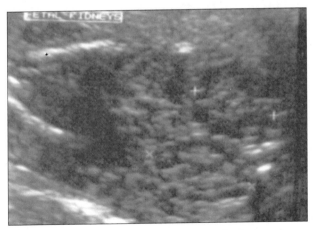

Fig. 11.26: Polycystic kidneys with severe oligohydramnios

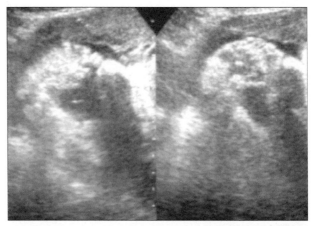

Fig. 11.27: Fetal foot turned medially in a case of clubfoot. Visualize the sole of the foot and if in this view you can see the tibia it is a clubfoot deformity. Clubfoot deformity can be associated with Trisomy 18, so a thorough check for stigmata of Trisomy 18 should be done

Firstly try and assess plenty of normal fetuses and gradually get into the habit of suspecting something abnormal. For any doubts open your textbook and never hesitate to give a differential diagnosis.

CHAPTER 12

Wellbeing in the
Third Trimester

1. Look for any hyperechoic areas in the placenta with or without shadowing as these indicate basal stippling (Fig. 12.1) and calcification (Fig. 12.2).
2. Assess the liquor amnii (Fig. 12.3) for any oligohydramnios (Fig. 12.4) as that changes the biophysical score and decides the mode and timing of termination of the pregnancy. Remember that if you have a color Doppler switch on the color to measure the pocket of liquor because many a times there is only cord in that pocket and it will give a wrong amniotic fluid index (Fig. 12.5).
3. Presentation of the fetus should always be mentioned. See whether the fetus is cephalic (Fig. 12.6) or breech (Fig. 12.7) (extended or footling or knee) or transverse (cranium in the right/left flank) or oblique (cranium in the right/left iliac fossa or in the right/left hypochondrium).
4. Always look for anomalies even in the third trimester.
5. Assess the fetal maturity. If you have previous reports especially the one in the first trimester (dating scan) it is

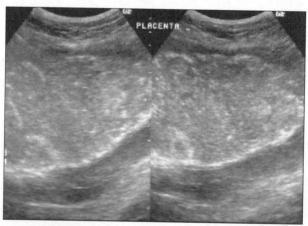

Fig. 12.1: Grade II placenta with basal stippling

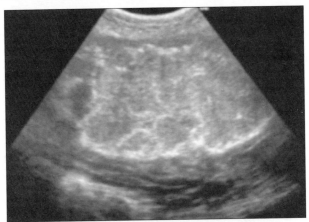

Fig. 12.2: Grade III placenta with calcification along the basal plate, chorionic plate and intercotyledons

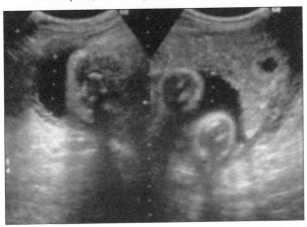

Fig. 12.3: Amniotic fluid index assessment. The uterus is divided into four quadrants by the midline and transverse axis and the amniotic fluid as the deepest vertical pocket free of fetal parts and umbilical cord is measured in each quadrant and all four quadrants add up to give the amniotic fluid index. Pregnancy of 38 weeks and 5 days with normal liquor amnii

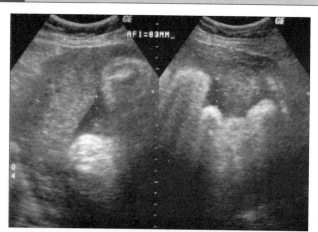

Fig. 12.4: Pregnancy of 37 weeks and 2 days with oligohydramnios

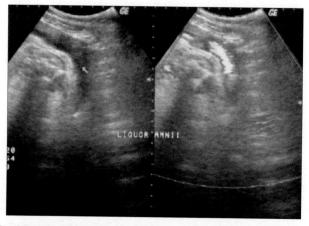

Fig. 12.5: Remember that if you have a color Doppler switch on the color to measure the pocket of liquor because many a times there is only cord in that pocket and it will give a wrong amniotic fluid index. Pocket which is full of umbilical cord so this pocket measurement is 0 mm not 28 mm as originally thought on a 2D image

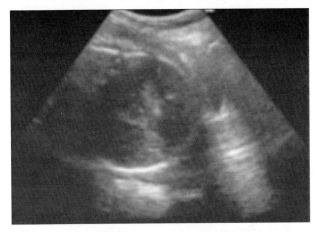

Fig. 12.6: Cephalic presentation with the cranium opposed to the cervix

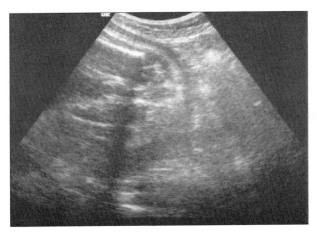

Fig. 12.7: Extended breech presentation with the fetal buttocks opposed to the cervix

always advisable to calculate the maturity according to that. If you are scanning the patient first time in the third trimester go in for multiple parameter evaluation for maturity evaluation like distal femoral epiphysis (Fig. 12.8), femoral length and cranial parameters.

6. Fetal biometry to be assessed for calculating the fetal weight. The parameters are:
   a. Biparietal diameter (Fig. 12.9)
   b. Occipitofrontal distance (Fig. 12.9)
   c. Head perimeter (Fig. 12.9)
   d. Abdominal perimeter (Fig. 12.10)
   e. Femoral length (Fig. 12.10)
   f. Fetal weight is calculated automatically by the machine depending on the formula one is using (Fig. 12.11).

7. Please remember that the EDD is calculated according to the fetal age (Fig. 12.11) (maturity) and not fetal size. Secondly during the pregnancy you cannot have a different EDD everytime you are scanning. Thirdly for different parameters you cannot have a different EDD.

8. One can look in for whether the umbilical cord is around the neck or not and how many loops. Even on a 2D (Fig. 12.12) one can always have a suspicion but it should always be confirmed by color flow mapping (Figs 12.13 and 12.14). The management or termination of pregnancy does not solely lie on the fact whether a loop of umbilical cord is around the neck or not. Other parameters for fetal wellbeing are detrimental for these.

9. In patients of previous cesarian the lower segment should be measured (Fig. 12.15). The bladder should be partially full and without applying pressure measure the myometrium and exclude the urinary bladder wall. It can be done by a transabdominal scan, transvaginal scan or a translabial scan.

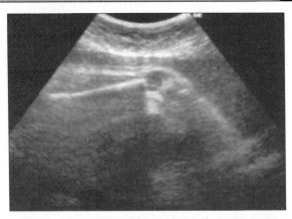

Fig. 12.8: The distal femoral epiphysis can be measured and maturity known as it starts appearing only after 35 weeks

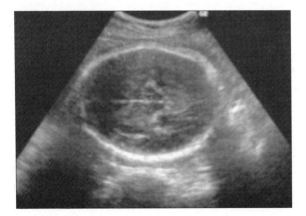

Fig. 12.9: Section for cranial biometry consisting of the thalamus, the third ventricle and the cavum septum pellucidum. The biparietal diameter is the side to side measurement from the outer table of the proximal skull to the inner table of the distal skull. The head perimeter is the the total cranial circumference, which includes the maximum anteroposterior diameter. The occipitofrontal diameter is the front to back measurement from the outer table on both sides

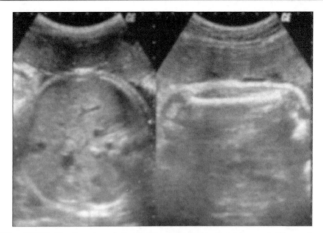

Fig. 12.10: Section for abdominal perimeter measurement. The spine should be posterior and the umbilical part of the portal vein anteriorly. Femoral length measurement for assessing fetal biometry

```
Ref MD:                    NOTE:
             POS:          PLAC:                        ← 1/2 ▮
MEASUREMENTS CUR  LAST      1       2      3      AGE        GP
BPD(HADLOCK)  u   84.6mm (  84.6            )  34W0D±3W1D  50%
HC(HADLOCK)   y   309mm  (  309             )  34W4D±3W0D  26%
OFD(HC)           112mm  (  112             )
AC(HADLOCK)   y   296mm  (  296             )  33W4D±3W0D  40%
FL(HADLOCK)   u   67.4mm (  67.4            )  34W5D±3W0D  58%
CRL(HADLOCK)  y          (                  )
GS(HELLMAN)   u          (                  )


  CALCULATIONS
CI     75.?(78-86)              EFW 2328g±349g ( 5lb  2oz)  44%
FL/BPD 79.7(71-87)             Based On:(BPD HC AC  FL      )
FL/AC  22.8(20-24)              AFI(cm)          HR(BPM)
FL/HC  21.0(19.4-21.8)   LMP:(OPE)23/11/02
HC/AC  1.046(0.95-1.11)  AGE: LMP 34W0D        CUA 34W0D
                         EDD: LMP 30/08/03     CUA 30/08/03
COMMENTS:
```

Fig. 12.11: The chart shows a fetal weight of 2328 grams for 34 weeks with an EDD of 30/08/03

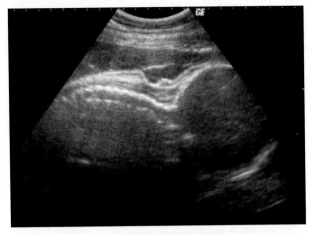

Fig. 12.12: Strong suspicion of two loops of
umbilical cord on a 2D image

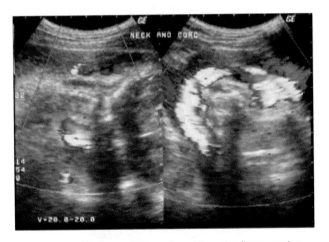

Fig. 12.13: Findings of 2D confirmed by color flow mapping
when these two loops are demonstrated

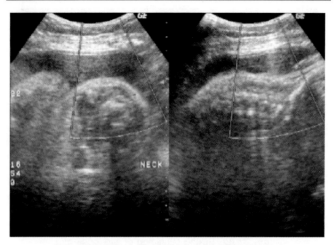

Fig. 12.14: No cord seen near or around the fetal neck as seen on color flow mapping

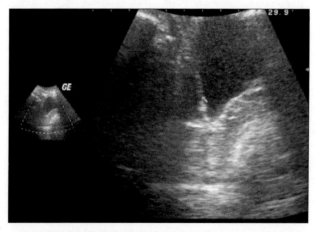

Fig. 12.15: Thinned lower segment scar seen in a patient of previous cesarian

10. These are the factors to see for the normalcy of the fetus and its environment. Then one has to go into details of assessing the fetus by biophysical scoring and color Doppler studies to check for the timing of termination of the pregnancy.

CHAPTER 13

Fetal Wellbeing by Biophysical Scoring and Color Doppler Studies

1. The biophysical score is a combination of Acute and Chronic markers. Liquor amnii reflects Chronic compromise and Non-stress test, Movements, Tone and Breathing Movements reflect Acute compromise. Each parameter is given a score out of 02 and then all are added up to take out a Biophysical Score of out of 10. Refer to your textbooks for scoring 0, 01 or 02 each and every parameter so as to decide the time and mode of delivery (Fig. 13.1).

2. Doppler ultrasound has given us a noninvasive method of evaluation of blood flow in the fetoplacental and uteroplacental circulation in normal and complicated pregnancies. The vessels that one requires to assess are :

   a. Main Uterine Arteries: Abnormal waveform has a notch in early diastole or a systolic notch or a Resistive Index of more than 0.55 or a major right to left variation (Figs 13.2 and 13.3).

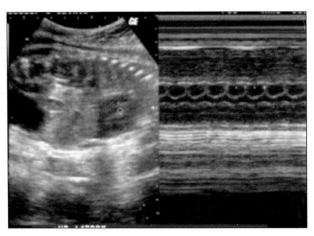

Fig. 13.1: The non-stress test is seen by checking the heart rate before and after fetal movements, to see whether there is any increase for a sufficient period of time or not

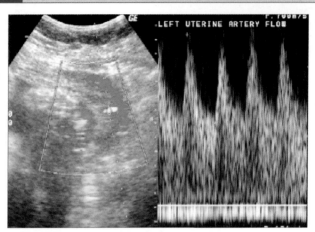

Fig. 13.2: Uterine arteries reflect trophoblastic invasion and the prediction of a hypertensive disorder in low risk mothers and perinatal morbidity and mortality in high risk mothers. Normal uterine artery flow with flow in diastole and a resistive index of less than 0.55 after 22 weeks

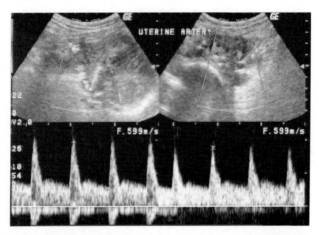

Fig. 13.3: Abnormal waveform showing a notch in early diastole. Other abnormal waveforms can have a systolic notch or a resistive index of more than 0.55 or a major right to left variation

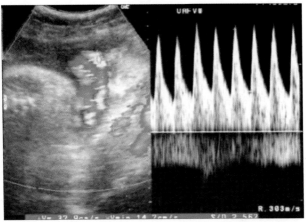

Fig. 13.4: Umbilical arteries reflect placental obliteration and one should have sufficient flow in diastole for a normal waveform

b. Umbilical Artery: Abnormal waveform has absent end diastolic flow or reversal of end diastolic flow (Figs 13.4 and 13.5).

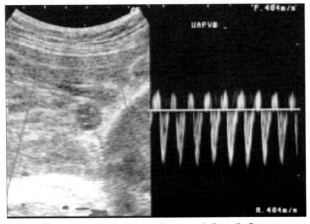

Fig. 13.5: Abnormal waveform has absent end diastolic flow or reversal of end diastolic flow. This waveform shows reversal of flow in diastole

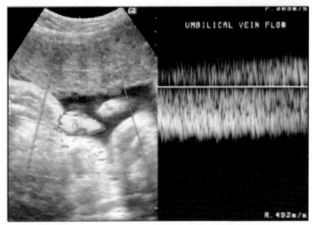

Fig. 13.6: Normal continuous flow in a umbilical vein flow
pattern and this reflects myocardial function

c. Umbilical Vein: Abnormal waveform has a double
pulsatile pattern (Figs 13.6 and 13.7).

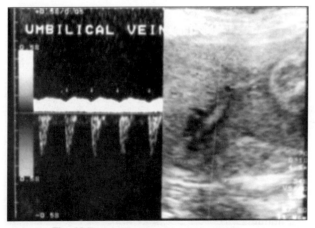

Fig. 13.7: Double pulsatile pattern seen in an
abnormal umbilical vein flow pattern

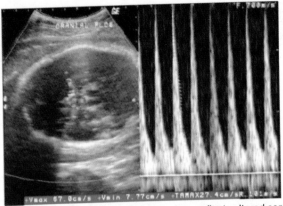

Fig. 13.8: The middle cerebral artery waveform reflects altered cerebral flow or cerebral edema. In hypoxia the blood flow to the middle cerebral artery increases as a reflex redistribution of fetal cardiac output. Normal waveform with a pulsatility index of 2.15

d. Middle Cerebral Artery: Abnormal waveform has decreased resistance which increases with continued hypoxia (Figs 13.8 and 13.9).

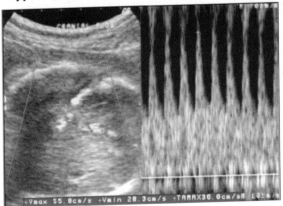

Fig. 13.9: Abnormal waveform with increased blood flow to the middle cerebral artery with a pulsatility index of 0.76

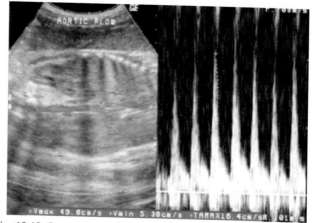

Fig. 13.10: Descending aorta reflects flow from the abdominal viscera and lower limbs. Normal waveform with adequate diastolic flow

    e. Descending Aorta: Abnormal waveform has a markedly reduced flow in diastole (Figs 13.10 and 13.11).

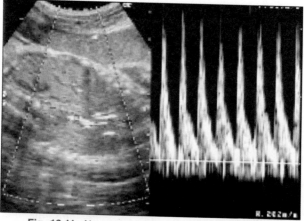

Fig. 13.11: Abnormal waveform with reduced flow in diastole for redistribution to other vital organs

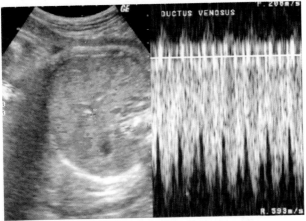

Fig. 13.12: Ductus venosus flow reflects acidosis.
Normal waveform with plenty of flow in diastole

f. Ductus Venosus: Abnormal waveform has an absent forward flow in diastole (Figs 13.12 and 13.13).

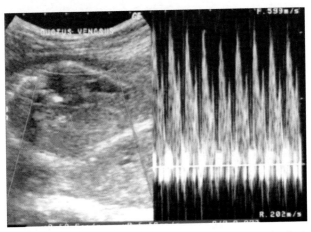

Fig. 13.13: Abnormal waveform with a reduced forward flow in diastole

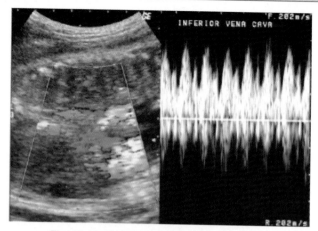

Fig. 13.14: Normal triphasic inferior vena cava
flow reflecting myocardial function

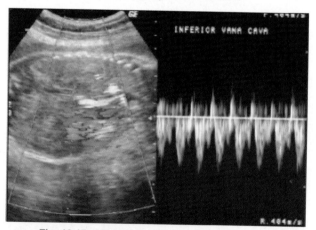

Fig. 13.15: Abnormal waveform with an increased
reversed flow in diastole

g. Inferior Vena Cava: Abnormal waveform has an increased
   reversed flow (Figs 13.14 and 13.15).

FETAL SURVEILLANCE OR FETAL WELLBEING

When to evaluate
1. Unexplained fetal death
2. Decreased fetal movements
3. Maternal chronic hypertension
4. Pre-eclampsia (PIH)
5. Maternal diabetes mellitus
6. Chronic renal disease
7. Cyanotic heart disease
8. Rh or other isoimmunization
9. Hemoglobinopathies
10. Immunological disorders
11. Oligohydramnios
12. Polyhydramnios
13. Intrauterine growth retardation
14. Multiple gestations
15. Post-dated pregnancy
16. Preterm labor
17. Premature rupture of membranes
18. History bleeding in first trimester
19. Elderly women
20. ART pregnancies

CHAPTER 14

Summary of Obstetric Scanning

1. Be careful and mention whatever you see.
2. Look for cardiac activity very carefully otherwise reassess.
3. Look for shape of gestational sac and size of yolk sac.
4. Look for placental site and fetal behavior.
5. Take the biometric measurements carefully and look for anything abnormal.
6. Look for fetal movements and Doppler flow to various organs in a stressed fetus.
7. Practise hard and look for normal status because there are plenty of normal physiological changes.
8. Just give plenty of time 13 days is nothing for learning Obstetrical Ultrasound, you require months and months of hard work.

CHAPTER 15

Normal Female Pelvis

Transabdominal and transvaginal scanning are two methods which complement each other and allow for a complete evaluation of the pelvic organs.

Evaluation of the normal female pelvis comprises of checking the pelvic viscera in detail and comprises of:

1. Uterus
   a. **Size:** Normal uterine size varies with age.
      i. The neonatal uterus is relatively large, with the body being larger than the cervix.
      ii. In early childhood the uterus has a tubular shape with the uterine body being smaller than the cervix (Fig. 15.1).
      iii. As the child approaches menarche, the uterine body again increases in size.
      iv. In the postmenarchal period, the body is typically twice the size of the cervix (Fig. 15.2). The dimensions of the normal uterus in women of childbearing age is $80 \times 40 \times 40$ mm. The multiparous uterus is larger than the nulliparous uterus by up to 10 mm in each dimension.
   b. **Divisions:** Fundus, body (Corpus) and cervix (Fig. 15.3). The body of the uterus is separated from the cervix by the isthmus at the level of the internal os. Variety of different positions in relation to the angle of the cervix to the vagina (version) and the angle of body of the uterus at the isthmus (flexion).The cervix is homogeneous in echotexture with a hypoechoic central canal.
   c. **Parts** (Fig. 15.4):
      i. *Endometrium*: It is visualized as a hyperechoic band in the center of the uterus. The total thickness of the endometrium represents the anterior and posterior opposed layers. When endometrial fluid is present,

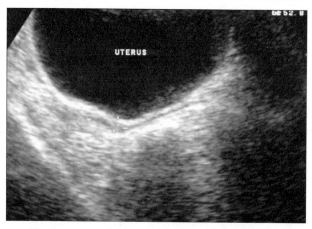

Fig. 15.1: Infantile uterus has a tubular shape with the uterine body being smaller than the cervix

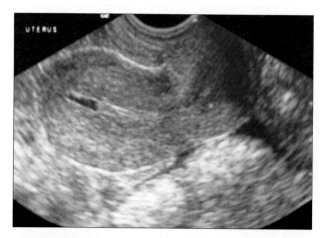

Fig. 15.2: In the postmenarchal period, the body is typically twice the size of the cervix. The dimensions of the normal uterus in women of childbearing age is 80 × 40 × 40 mm

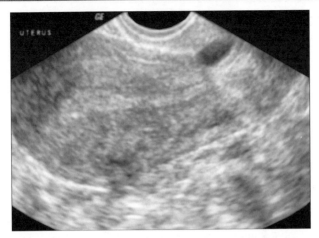

Fig. 15.3: The uterus has a fundus, body (Corpus) and cervix

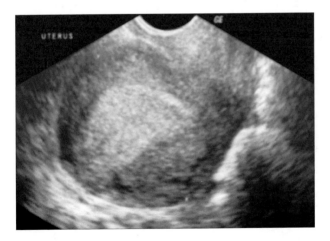

Fig. 15.4: The uterus has an *endometrium* which is visualized as a hyperechoic band in the center of the uterus and myometrium which should be homogeneous with smooth margins

this should not be included in the endometrial thickness, measurement. Normal endometrial thickness and appearance varies with the phase of the menstrual cycle.

ii. *Myometrium*: The myometrium should be homogeneous with smooth margins.

2. Fallopian Tube: The normal fallopian tube is difficult to distinguish from surrounding vessels and ligaments. It usually is not visualized unless abnormal or surrounded by fluid.

3. Ovaries

   a. **Size:** Ovaries in girls younger than 2 years of age are typically less than 1 ml in volume, although in neonates they can be slightly larger. The ovaries increase in size in prepubertal girls (Fig. 15.5) with follicles up to 1 cm in size. After menarche, the ovaries are ovoid in shape and generally measure 30 × 20 × 20 mm (Fig. 15.6).

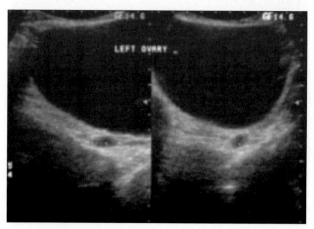

Fig. 15.5: Ovaries in a prepubertal female

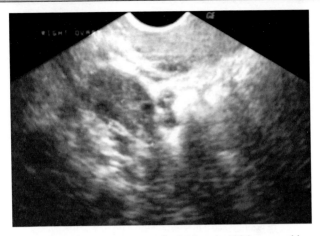

Fig. 15.6: Ovaries in a postpubertal female which are ovoid in shape and generally measure 30 × 20 × 20 mm

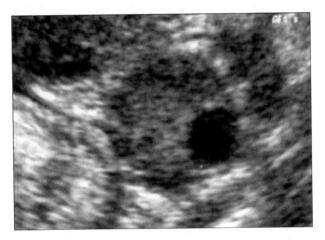

Fig. 15.7: In the proliferative phase of the menstrual cycle, multiple small follicles are visualized, usually 10 mm in diameter or less. Small 07 mm follicle seen on the 8th day of the cycle

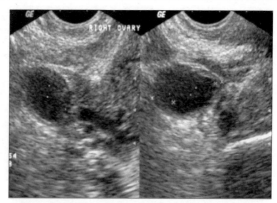

Fig. 15.8: The follicle increases in size and a 16 mm maturing follicle is seen on the 11th day of the cycle

b. Folliculogenesis: In the proliferative phase of the menstrual cycle, multiple small follicles are visualized, usually 10 mm in diameter or less (Fig. 15.7). A dominant follicle develops (Fig. 15.8) in the midcycle, which measures up to 20 mm in diameter (Fig. 15.9). After ovulation, the corpus luteum cyst develops (Fig. 15.10).

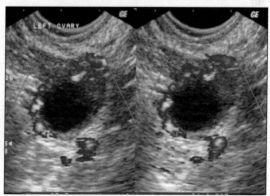

Fig. 15.9: A dominant follicle is seen in the midcycle, which measures 19 mm in diameter

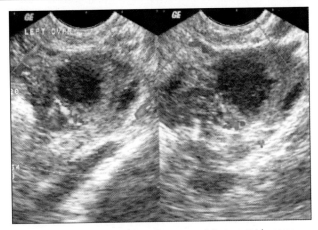

Fig. 15.10: After ovulation, the corpus luteum cyst is seen as a hypoechoic area within the ovary

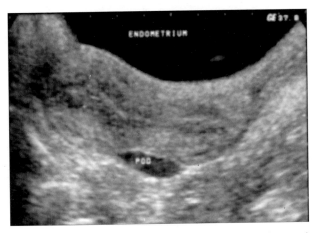

Fig. 15.11: A small amount of fluid is present in the cul-de-sac of asymptomatic women throughout the menstrual cycle

4. Pouch of Douglas: A small amount of fluid is present in the cul-de-sac of asymptomatic women throughout the menstrual cycle (Fig. 15.11).

   Remember whenever you see any pathology you are supposed to be mentioning the size, echo pattern, if possible mobility, if you have a color Doppler the vascularity and the organ of origin of the lesion. Do not tend to give a histopathological diagnosis because there are so many overlaps.

CHAPTER 16

Uterine Disorders

1. Myometrium
   a. Fibroids: (Table 16.1)
      i. Fibroids are described by their location. They can be submucosal (Fig. 16.1) (displacing/distorting the endometrium), intramural (Fig. 16.2) (within the wall of the uterus and not distorting either the endometrial cavity or the uterine contour), subserosal (Fig. 16.3) (seen distorting the uterine contour), panmural (Fig. 16.4) (through and through from the outer surface till the endometrial cavity) or pedunculated (Fig. 16.5).
      ii. Fibroids can undergo atrophic, hyaline (irregular anechoic areas in the fibroid with no distal acoustic enhancement) (Fig. 16.6), cystic (Fig. 16.7) (irregular anechoic areas in the fibroid with distal acoustic enhancement), myxomatous, lipomatous, calcific (high level echoes within the fibroid with distal acoustic shadowing) and carneous degeneration and infarction, infection, torsion and malignant change.
   b. Adenomyosis: (Figs 16.8 and 16.9) The sonographic features are an enlarged, globular and bosselated uterus with thickening, and focal or diffuse speckled appearance of the myometrium.
   c. Obstruction: Patients with hydrocolpos (fluid in the vagina) and hydrometrocolpos (fluid in the vagina and uterus) (Fig. 16.10) usually are seen soon after birth or at puberty when secretions cause obstruction because of an intact hymen or vaginal atresia. Hematometra is also seen in patients with cervical cancer or cervical stenosis (Fig. 16.11).
   d. Uterine calcifications: The most common cause of dense echoes in the uterus are calcifications resulting from

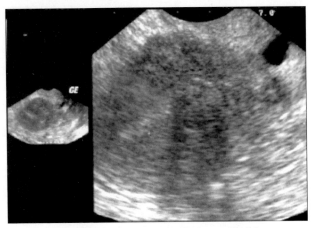

Fig. 16.1: Posterior wall submucous fibroid
(displacing/distorting the endometrium)

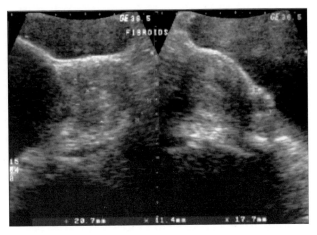

Fig. 16.2: Two right wall interstitial fibroids. (within the wall
of the uterus and not distorting either the endometrial
cavity or the uterine contour)

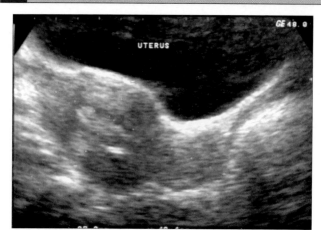

Fig. 16.3: Anterior wall and posterior wall subserous fibroids. (seen distorting the uterine contour)

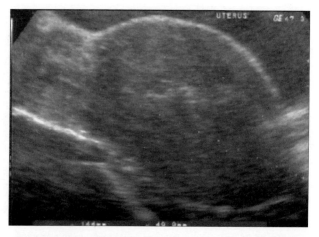

Fig. 16.4: Anterior wall panmural fibroid. (through and through from the outer surface till the endometrial cavity)

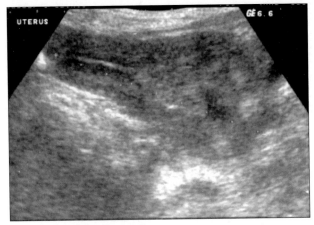

Fig. 16.5: Pedunculated fibroid seen in the uterine
corpus and through the cervical canal

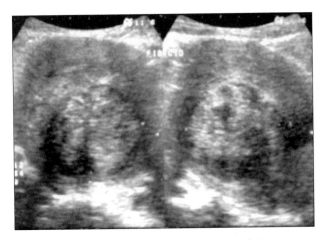

Fig. 16.6: Hyaline degeneration (irregular anechoic areas
in the fibroid with no distal acoustic enhancement)
in a posterior wall panmural fibroid

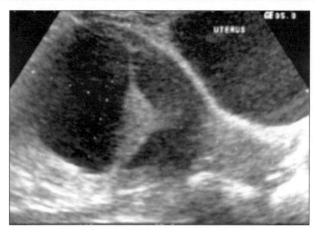

Fig. 16.7: Cystic degeneration (irregular anechoic areas in the fibroid with distal acoustic enhancement) in a fundal panmural fibroid

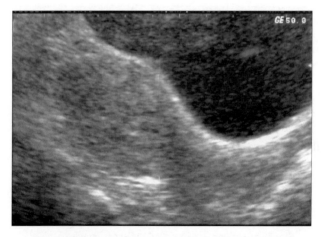

Fig. 16.8: Adenomyotic uterus with a diffuse speckled appearance of the myometrium

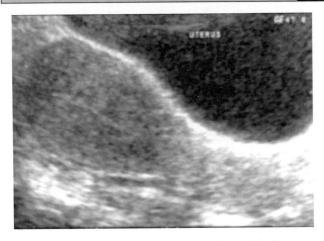

Fig. 16.9: An enlarged, globular and bosselated adenomyotic uterus

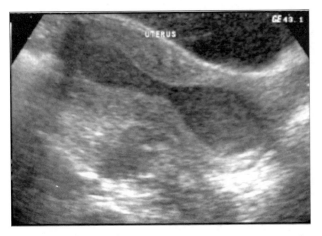

Fig. 16.10: Hydrometrocolpos (fluid in the vagina and uterus) seen at puberty when secretions cause obstruction because of an intact hymen or vaginal atresia

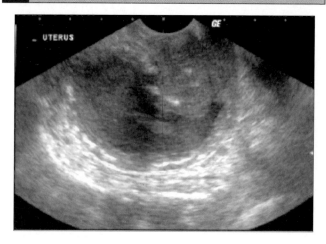

Fig. 16.11: Hematometra seen in patients with cervical cancer. Note the atrophic myometrium with calcific foci

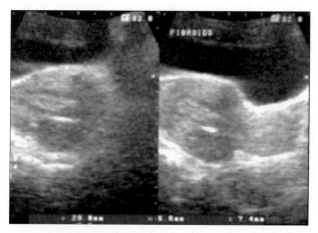

Fig. 16.12: Dense echoes in the uterus from calcifications resulting from fibroids

fibroids (Fig. 16.12). A less common cause of calcification within the uterus is that of the arcuate artery calcification.

2. Endometrium

   a. Endometritis: Endometritis occurs in association with pelvic inflammatory disease and in postpartum patients. The endometrium appears echogenic (Fig. 16.13) or irregular with a small amount of endometrial fluid.

   b. Synechiae: Vaginal sonography may demonstrate bright echoes within the endometrial cavity in this condition.

   c. Endometrial hyperplasia, polyps, and cancer

      i. Endometrial hyperplasia usually occurs secondary to the trophic influence of unopposed estrogen; the endometrium is thickened either diffusely or focally (Fig. 16.14).

      ii. Endometrial polyps usually are asymptomatic (Figs 16.15 and 16.16) but may cause uterine bleeding. They also cause diffuse or focal endometrial thickening. In both of these conditions (endometrial hyperplasia and polyps), the interface between the endometrium and the myometrium is preserved.

      iii. Endometrial cancer also is a cause endometrial thickening. The diagnosis is suggested when there is loss of the endometrial-myometrial interface (Figs 16.17 and 16.18). Sonography is helpful in assessing superficial and deep invasion and for follow-up management.

   d. Endometrial fluid: Fluid within the endometrial cavity is seen in both normal and pathologic conditions. In women in the menstrual phase of their cycle, a tiny amount of fluid is a normal finding. Fluid within the endometrium is also seen in normal early pregnancy and abnormal pregnancy (missed abortion, ectopic

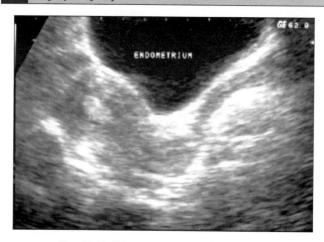

Fig. 16.13: Echogenic irregular endometrium because of endometritis

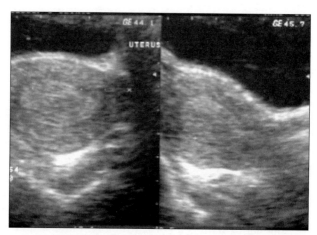

Fig. 16.14: Diffusely thickened endometrium

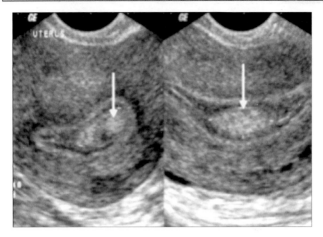

Fig. 16.15: Endometrial polyp causing a focal endometrial thickening in a patient of intermenstrual spotting

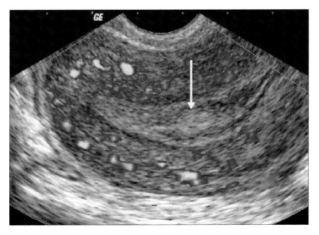

Fig. 16.16: Patient of menometrorrhagia with an echogenic endometrial polyp. Note that the interface between the endometrium and the myometrium is preserved

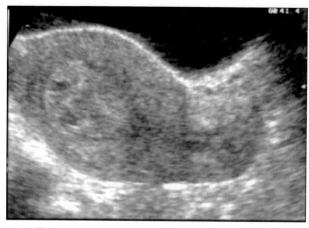

Fig. 16.17: Thickened inhomogeneous endometrium with multiple interspersed cystic spaces

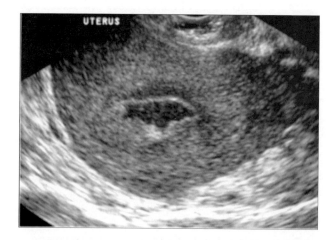

Fig. 16.18: Thickened endometrium with a fluid collection and a loss of the endometrial-myometrial interface at the posterior aspect

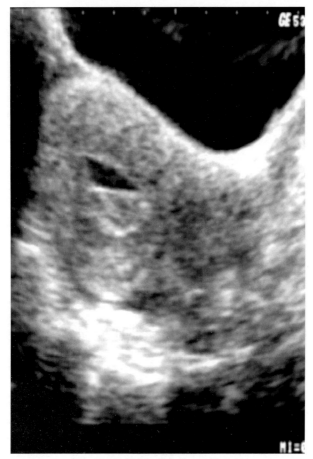

Fig. 16.19: Fluid within the cavity with a focal echogenic area

pregnancy, and molar pregnancy). Other causes of endometrial fluid include infection and obstruction. In older patients, fluid can be secondary to malignancy [uterine (Fig. 16.19), cervical, tubal, or ovarian];

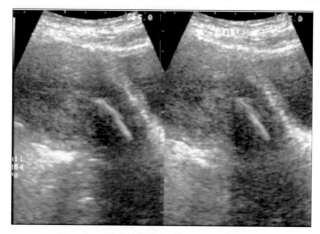

Fig. 16.20: Intrauterine contraceptive device
seen in the uterine corpus

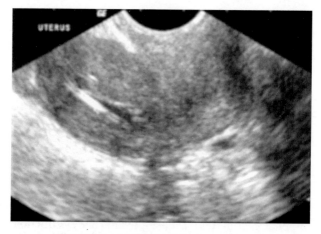

Fig. 16.21: Intrauterine contraceptive device
seen in the uterine fundus

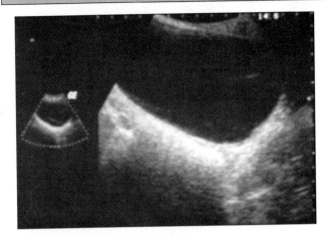

Fig. 16.22: A very small uterine anlage in a case of primary amenorrhea

however, cervical stenosis of a benign etiology (especially in women who previously had children or instrumentation) is more common. The presence of fever in a woman with a fluid collection suggests pyometra.

e. Intrauterine contraception devices: Another cause of bright reflectors within the uterus is intrauterine contraceptive devices (Figs 16.20 and 16.21). Ultrasound is helpful in locating the intrauterine contraceptive device when the string cannot be felt. Ultrasound is used to precisely locate the position of the intrauterine contraceptive device relative to the endometrial lumen and surrounding myometrium.

3. Shape and size: One can see a small hypoplastic uterus or an uterine anlage in much older females (Fig. 16.22).

Table 16.1: Sonographic evaluation of fibroids

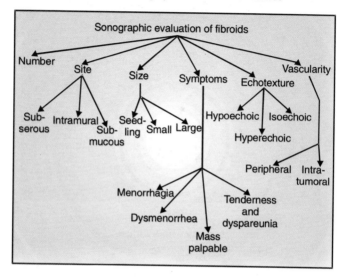

CHAPTER 17

Ovarian Disorders

The differential diagnosis of an ovarian disorder largely depends on factors such as patient's age, time since last menstrual period, symptoms, pregnancy test result, any prior surgery, and findings on examination.

Adnexal masses on ultrasound are labeled as completely cystic, complex (mixed cystic and solid), or solid.

1. Anechoic cysts/cystic lesions: Anechoic cysts are thin-walled, and show distal acoustic enhancement and are unlikely to be malignant.

   a. Functional cysts (Fig. 17.1) are most common anechoic cysts. These are usually small and measure less than 2 cm in diameter; but may even measure up to 10 cm. They usually regress spontaneously and should be followed up after the next period.

   b. Paraovarian cysts: Paraovarian cysts (Fig. 17.2) arise from the broad ligament. They do not show any change during the menstrual cycle.

   c. Theca lutein cysts: Theca lutein cysts are large ovarian cysts usually bilateral and can appear as multiloculated masses. They are most commonly associated with gestational trophoblastic disease but can also be secondary to infertility drugs and multiple gestations.

2. Complex cysts: They contain both fluid and solid areas and can be predominantly solid or cystic.

   a. Endometriosis: In women of menstrual age, the most common etiology of a complex ovarian cyst is hemorrhagic cyst. Diffuse low-level echoes seen in the cystic mass are characteristic of a "chocolate cyst" (Figs 17.3 and 17.4).

   b. Tubo-ovarian abscess: Inhomogeneous mass with the ovary and tube seen engulfed within it. Usually bilateral (Figs 17.5 and 17.6).

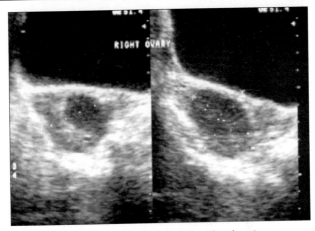

Fig. 17.1: Simple anechoic functional cyst

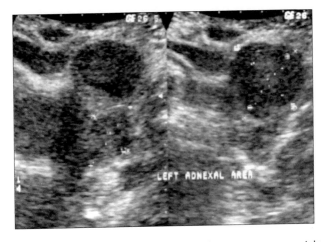

Fig. 17.2: Left paraovarian cyst with the left ovary seen separately and the extraovarian cyst which is thin-walled seen separately

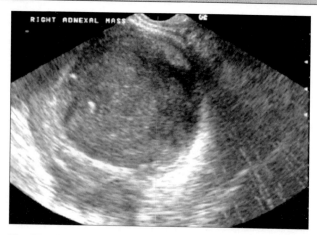

Fig. 17.3: Multiple diffuse fine echoes seen in this endometrioma

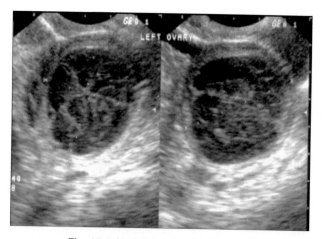

Fig. 17.4: Hemorrhagic cyst with dense coarse internal echoes

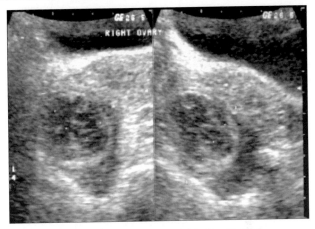

Fig. 17.5: Inhomogeneous right adnexal mass

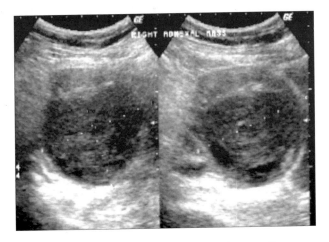

Fig. 17.6: Inhomogeneous right adnexal mass with
neither the ovary nor the tube seen separately

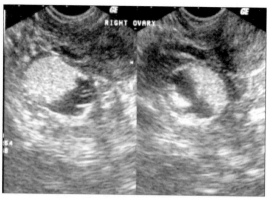

Fig. 17.7: Right ovarian dermoid

c. Dermoids: They have a spectrum of sonographic appearances including a completely cystic mass, a cystic mass with an echogenic mural-nodule, a fat-fluid level, echogenic foci with shadowing (teeth or bone), or a complex mass with internal septations and bright linear echoes (Figs 17.7 and 17.8).

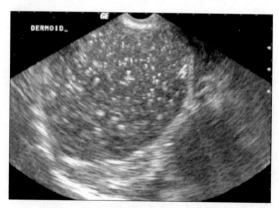

Fig. 17.8: Large dermoid with punctate hyperechoic foci

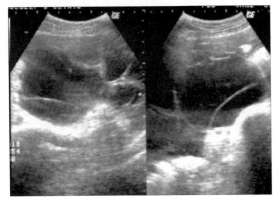

Fig. 17.9: Anechoic ovarian mass with multiple thin-septae

d. Ovarian neoplasms: The cystadenoma and cystadenocarcinoma are the most common types of epithelial tumors. Serous tumors are usually anechoic with septations (Fig. 17.9) and mucinous tumors usually have internal debris (Fig. 17.10). Thick septae, irregular solid areas (Fig. 17.11), ill- defined margins (Fig. 17.12) and ascites increase the likelihood of malignancy.

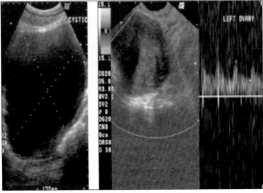

Fig. 17.10: Ovarian mass with multiple internal echoes

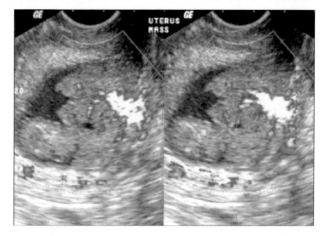

Fig. 17.11: Mass with solid areas and moderate vascularity

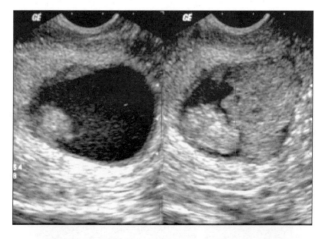

Fig. 17.12: Ill-defined mass within the cystic area
and coarse internal echoes

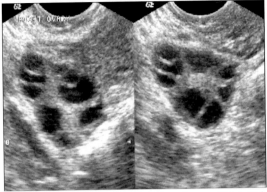

Fig. 17.13: Polycystic ovaries with a dense stroma and multiple thin-walled clear cysts along the periphery

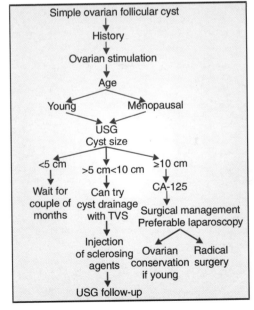

Fig. 17.14: Simple ovarian follicular cyst

e. Polycystic ovaries: Polycystic ovarian disease (infertility, hirsutism, obesity and oligomenorrhea), is one of the most common endocrine disorders. Sonographically, the ovaries are normal or enlarged with multiple small peripheral cysts, less than 8 mm in diameter with accompanying stromal hypertrophy (Figs 17.13 and 17.14).

3. Solid ovarian masses: Malignant ovarian neoplasms are the most common solid masses. The benign ovarian neoplasms, fibromas, thecomas and Brenner tumors also appear solid but are very uncommon.

CHAPTER 18

Miscellaneous Disorders of Female Pelvis

1. Cervical Disorders: The most common mass within the cervix is the nabothian cyst (Fig. 18.1). Solid masses include fibroids and malignancies. Cervical fibroids are hypoechoic and typically well defined, whereas cervical cancer is more likely to have ill-defined margins (Fig. 18.2).
2. Abnormal Vagina: The most common lesions visualized with sonography are Gartner's duct cysts (Fig. 18.3).
3. Abnormal Fallopian Tube: The major cause of fallopian tube abnormalities are infection and ectopic pregnancy.Old infection presents as an hydrosalpinx (Fig. 18.4) (a thin/thick-walled fluid-filled tubular structure). When an acute infection is present, the tube wall is thickened and hyperemic and internal debris (pyosalpinx) can be present. Normally a fallopian tube is seldom visible (Fig. 18.5).
4. Pouch of Douglas: One can find fluid in the POD mostly in cases of infection (Fig. 18.6).

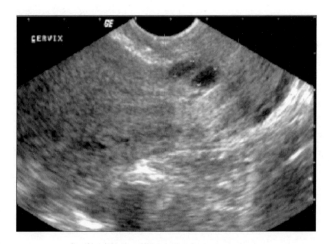

Fig. 18.1: Multiple ectatic endocervical glands seen in the cervix

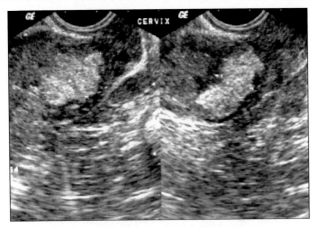

Fig. 18.2: Inhomogeneous ill-defined mass seen
in the left wall of the cervix

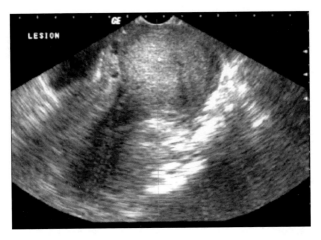

Fig. 18.3: Large mass seen in the vagina

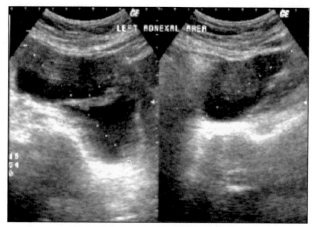

Fig. 18.4: Left hydrosalpinx with the
left ovary seen separately

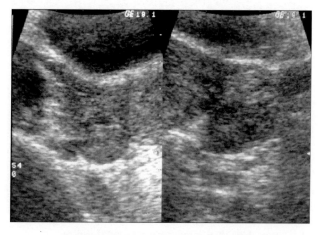

Fig. 18.5: Normal fallopian tubes seen

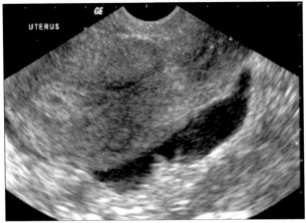

Fig. 18.6: Fluid in the pouch of Douglas seen in a case of acute pelvic inflammatory disease

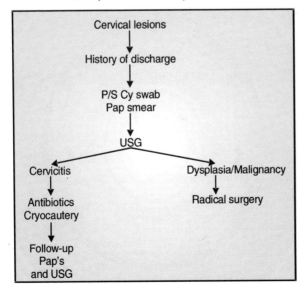

Fig. 18.7: Cervical lesions

In your reporting the salient features that require to be mentioned are:

1. Uterus: Size
2. Endometrium: Thickness and morphology. Any focal abnormality to be mentioned with size and echo pattern.
3. Myometrium: Echo pattern and presence of fibroids and their location.
4. Ovaries: Size (all three dimensions with total volume) and echo pattern. Any abnormality to be mentioned in terms of size, echo pattern, walls and focal abnormalities within it.
5. Extraovarian Adnexal Areas: Report whether any mass is delineated or not.
6. Free fluid or fluid loculi in the pouch of Douglas or adnexa.

CHAPTER 19

Ultrasound, Color Doppler and 3D Ultrasound for Assessment of an Infertile Female

1. Transvaginal sonography has an important role in the management of infertility.
2. Anovulation and ovulatory dysfunction are important factors in the etiology of infertility.
3. In addition the correct prediction or timing of ovulation is critical for infertility therapies such as intrauterine insemination, artificial or therapeutic insemination using donor sperm and the timing of intercourse during ovulation induction therapies.

2D EVALUATION (Figs 19.1 to 19.7)

Confirming Ovulation

1. Disappearance of the follicle is noted in 91 percent of cases after ovulation and a decrease in follicle size occurs in another 9 percent.
2. Other signs suggesting that ovulation has occurred are the appearance of cul-de-sac fluid, particularly when it was not present in a previous scan, or the development of intrafollicular eachoes suggesting the formation of a hemorrhagic corpus luteum.

Ovary in Anovulatory Cycles

1. In an anovulatory cycle, ultrasound imaging of the ovaries will reveal either a lack of any follicular development, particularly in the hypogonadotropic hypogonadal patient.
2. A dominant follicle larger than 16 mm in diameter will not develop.
3. Anovulation can be diagnosed when serial scans do not show development of a follicle.

Endometrium

1. The endometrial cavity should be visualized as a separate entity within the uterus in virtually all menstruating patients.

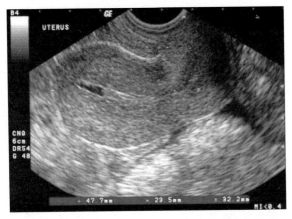

Fig. 19.1: Days 2: Baseline ultrasound shows a homogeneous myometrium, small endometrial fluid collection and a thin endometrium with no focal lesions

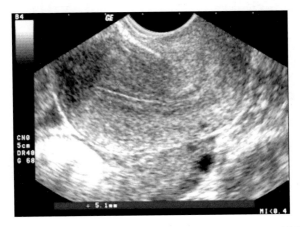

Fig. 19.2: Days 6: The endometrium is trilayered and 05 mm thick

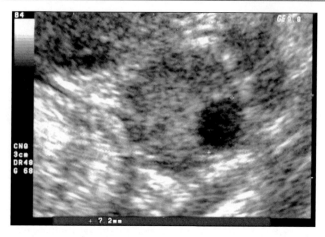

Fig. 19.3: Days 6: The left ovary shows a 07 mm follicle

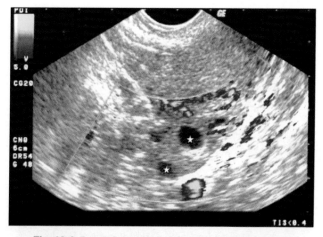

Fig. 19.4: Day 6: Stimulated cycle with multiple immature follicles (stars) seen in the ovary

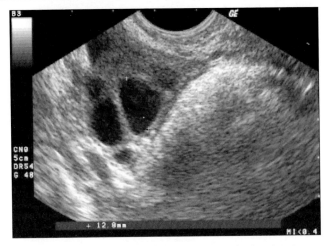

Fig. 19.5: Day 9: Multiple follicles seen in a stimulated cycle.
Largest of these measures 13 mm across

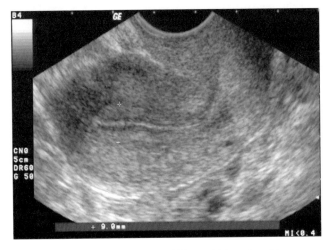

Fig. 19.6: Days 10: Trilayered 09 mm thick endometrium

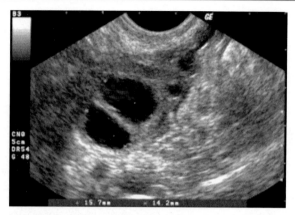

Fig. 19.7: Days 10: Multiple follicles seen with the largest measuring up to 16 mm across in the right ovary

2. The cyclic changes of the endometrium can be imaged using transvaginal ultrasound during the different phases of the menstrual cycle.
3. The hormonal and ovulatory status of the patients can be assessed by evaluating the endometrial patterns.

Early Proliferative Phase

1. The anechoic central echo noted during early menses is replaced by a hyperechoic central line and the endometrium begins to thicken, forming the three-line sign.
2. In the follicular phase, the halo which is about 2 mm thick and surrounds the endometrium, is present. There is no posterior enhancement.

Late Proliferative Phase

1. There is continued thickening of the endometrial echo complex in the late proliferative phase.
2. The halo is still present.

3. The endometrial complex is still imaged as three parallel lines, but the outer lines may begin to thicken.
4. The total endometrial thickness increases and may reach 09-10 mm or greater in total thickness.
5. There is no posterior enhancement.

Luteal Phase

1. In the luteal phase the endometrium is thickened and is imaged as a homogeneous hyperechoic density with posterior enhancement and loss of the surrounding halo.
2. The three-line sign is gone.
3. The rate of increase of thickness slows and the endometrial echo complex soon achieves its greater anterior posterior dimension.
4. The echogenicity of the endometrium becomes hyper-echoic.

Minimally Stimulated or Single Line Endometrium

1. Patients with low oestrogen or excess androgen have generally have a single line endometrium similar to a late menstrual endometrium.

Endometrial Motion

1. The endometrium can be seen to move during real-time ultrasonographic imaging.
2. The movement can be quite impressive when first seen.

COLOR DOPPLER EVALUATION
(Figs 19.8 to 19.17)

1. Color Doppler sonology is a noninvasive technology to investigate the circulatory changes within the uterus and ovaries during different phases of the menstrual cycle.

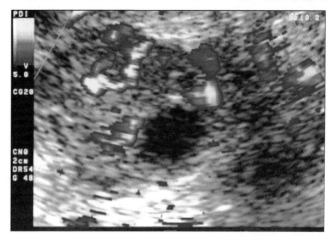

Fig. 19.8: Same follicle as in Figure 19.3 showing a
25 percent perifollicular vascularization

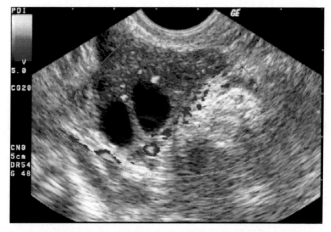

Fig. 19.9: Same follicles as in Figure 19.5 showing
a 25 percent perifollicular vascularization

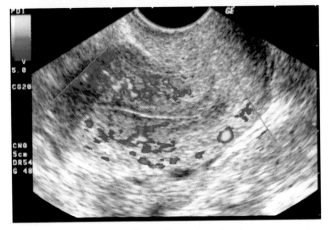

Fig. 19.10: The endometrium showing
a subendometrial vascularization

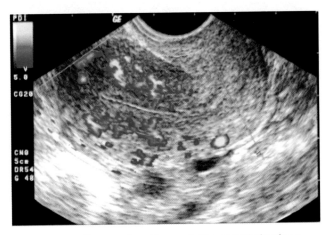

Fig. 19.11: Same endometrium as in Figure 19.6 showing a
subendometrial, basal layer and mid-zone vascularization

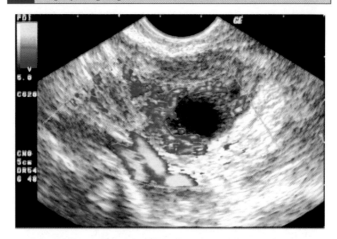

Fig. 19.12: Same follicles as in Figure 19.7 showing
a 50 percent perifollicular vascularization

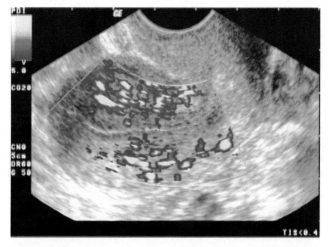

Fig. 19.13: Endometrium 10 mm thick and pre-ovulatory showing a
subendometrial, basal layer, mid-zone, inner layer and cavity vascularization

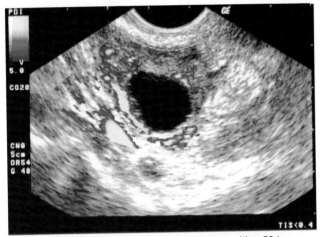

Fig. 19.14: Mature follicle, 19 mm across with a 50 to 75 percent perifollicular vascularization

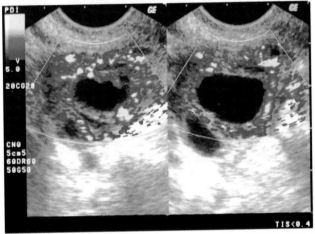

Fig. 19.15: Multiple follicles 18 to 21 mm across with a 50 to 75 percent perifollicular vascularization. More than 50 percent perifollicular vascularity is indicative of an increase in the number of mature oocytes recovered and higher fertilization rates than otherwise

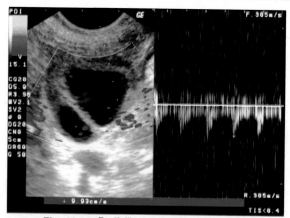

Fig. 19.16: Perifollicular vascularization with a peak systolic velocity around 10 cm/sec

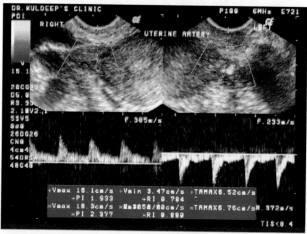

Fig. 19.17: If the uterine artery flow velocity waveform has a pulsatility index greater than 3.0 on the day of ovulation so the chances of a favorable outcome are extremely less. In this case the right uterine artery flow velocity waveform shows a pulsatility index of 1.93 and the left uterine artery flow velocity waveform shows a pulsatility index of 2.37

Physiological Changes of Menstrual Cycle by Color Doppler

1. It is very important to know the vascular changes in the menstrual cycle for the evaluation of female infertility.
2. It provides important information about blood flow to the maturing follicle, the vascular supply of the endometrium and corpus luteum vascularization which are very important for a successful outcome.

Endometrial Changes

1. The chances of implantation are dependent on endometrial receptivity and uterine vascular supply.
2. Endometrial vascularization as assessed by color flow mapping and duplex Doppler especially power Doppler is categorized as subendometrial, basal layer, mid zone and inner layer, and, cavity vascularization.
3. The deeper the vascularization noted, the better the outcome.
4. Failure of visualization of vascularization into and beyond the basal layer is associated with a uniformly poor outcome.
5. The uterine artery flow velocity waveform (bilateral) has a Resistive Index of 0.88 +/– 0.04 in the proliferative phase and starts decreasing as ovulation approaches.
6. The recent studies state that if the uterine artery flow velocity waveform has a Pulsatility Index greater than 3.0 on the day of ovulation then the chances of a favorable outcome are extremely less.

Ovarian Vascularity

1. The dominant follicle within the ovary is detected by a ring of angiogenesis around the follicle, which becomes more marked with increase in follicular size.

2. Vascular perfusion of maturing follicles has been graded on the percentage of follicular circumference seen to be vascularised using color flow mapping and power Doppler. The gradations are as follows:
   - Grade 1 is <25%
   - Grade 2 is < 50%
   - Grade 3 is < 75% and
   - Grade 4 is >75%.

3. More than 50 percent perifollicular vascularity is indicative of an increase in the number of mature oocytes recovered and higher fertilization rates than otherwise.

4. The peak systolic velocity is again an excellent marker to assess the chances of obtaining mature oocytes and therefore high grade preimplantation embryos.

Ovarian Stromal Blood Flow

1. Patients with a peak systolic velocity of more than 10 cm/second in the ovarian stromal arteries produce significantly higher mature oocytes and a higher pregnancy rate.

3D EVALUATION

1. HSG provides a good outline of the uterine cavity, it gives no information about the outer uterine contour.

2. Therefore, the distinction between different types of lateral fusion disorders in impossible.

3. Definite diagnosis can be made noninvasively with 3D ultrasound.

4. The fundal cleft and the length of septum can be accurately measured by 3D ultrasound and allow accurate differential diagnosis between an accurate, subseptate and bicornuate uterus.

5. 3D three-planer image of a normal uterus is having a convex fundus and straight upper line of the uterine cavity.

6. An arcuate uterus has a convex fundus but concave rounded upperline of the uterine cavity.

7. A septate uterus is identified by a septum dividing the proximal portion of the uterine cavity but the uterine fundus is convex or with a shallow cleft (< 1 cm).

8. A bicornuate uterus has two well-formed cornua separated by a large fundus indentation (> 1 cm).

Normal Values

NUCHAL TRANSLUCENCY

- Nuchal translucency thickness usually increases with gestational age.
- 1.5 mm and 2.5 mm are the 50th and 95th percentile respectively for gestational ages between 10 and 12 weeks.
- 2.0 mm and 3.0 mm are the 50th and 95th percentile respectively for gestational ages between 12 and 14 weeks.

NUCHAL SKIN FOLD

- (14-18 weeks : Normal value < 04 mm, borderline 04-05 mm and > 05 mm requires further karyotypic analysis).
- (18-22 weeks : Normal value < 05 mm, borderline 05-06 mm and > 06 mm requires further karyotypic analysis).
- After 22 weeks the sensitivity of nuchal skin fold thickness measurement for predicting karyotypic abnormalities is poor.

RENAL PELVIS

- The values for the anteroposterior diameter of the renal pelvis (measured on a transverse view through the kidney).
- From 15-20 weeks of gestation < 04 mm is normal, 04-07 mm is borderline and > 08 mm is abnormal or hydronephrotic.
- From 20 weeks onwards < 06 mm is normal, 06-09 is borderline and > 10mm is abnormal or hydronephrotic.
- Borderline cases are to be reviewed by serial scans before labelling them as hydronephrotic. Check for caliectasis or ureteric dilatation.

VENTRICULAR ATRIUM

- The width of the body, anterior horn and posterior horn of the lateral ventricle are taken.
- (Normal value < 08 mm, borderline 08-10 mm and > 10 mm abnormal).

VENTRICULAR ATRIUM

- When the choroid plexus does not occupy the whole of the body of the lateral ventricle see for the measurement of the medial separation of the choroid plexus from the wall of the lateral ventricle.
- (Normal value < 02 mm, borderline 02-03 mm and > 03 mm is abnormal).

CEREBELLAR TRANSVERSE DIAMETER

The CTD in mm from 14-22 weeks is equal to the gestational age of the fetus in weeks.

CISTERNA MAGNA

(Normal value < 08 mm, borderline 08-10 mm and > 10 mm abnormal).

SMALL BOWEL

Small bowel segments usually are less than 07 mm in diameter.

LARGE BOWEL

A large bowel segment which is more than 20 mm wide near term can be termed as abnormal.

PERICARDIAL FLUID

Minimal pericardial fluid is a normal finding after 20 weeks of gestation. So pericardial fluid of more than 02 mm is regarded as abnormal.

CUTANEOUS THICKNESS

Subcutaneous edema is diagnosed as abnormal when it measures more than 05 mm.

APPENDIX 2

Measurement Methodology

AMNIOTIC FLUID INDEX ASSESSMENT

The uterus is divided into four quadrants by the midline and transverse axis and the amniotic fluid as the deepest vertical pocket free of fetal parts and umbilical cord is measured in each quadrant and all four quadrants add up to give the amniotic fluid index.

CHOROID PLEXUS

Choroid plexus occupies the whole of the body of the lateral ventricle. The anterior horn, body and posterior horn of the lateral ventricle should be measured. Measurement of any medial separation of the choroids plexus with the lateral ventricular wall should also be assessed for.

CEREBELLUM

The cerebellum is seen as a 'W' turned 90 degrees. The cerebellar hemispheres and the cerebellar vermis should be appreciated for posterior cranial fossa abnormalities. The cerebellar transverse diameter (CTD) is measured from the edges of both cerebellar hemispheres.

CISTERNA MAGNA

The cisterna magna is seen posterior to the cerebellar vermis and anterior to the occipital bone.

NUCHAL TRANSLUCENCY

The translucency (subcutaneous) between the skin and soft tissue posterior to the cervical spine has to be measured.

NUCHAL SKIN

The nuchal skin fold is measured from the posterior edge of the occipital bone and it includes the skin and the sonolucent area between the occipital bone and skin. Look in for any focal or diffuse thickening with/without septations.

CRANIAL BIOMETRY

Section for cranial biometry consists of the thalamus, the third ventricle and the cavum septum pellucidum.

- Biparietal diameter: Side to side measurement from the outer table of the proximal skull to the inner table of the distal skull.
- Head perimeter: The total cranial circumference, which includes the maximum anteroposterior diameter.
- Occipitofrontal diameter: Front to back measurement from the outer table on both sides.

ORBITAL MEASUREMENTS

- Ocular diameter: Measured from medial inner to medial lateral wall of the long orbit.
- Interocular distance: Measured from medial inner wall of one orbit to medial inner wall of the other orbit.
- Binocular distance: Measured from lateral inner wall of one orbit to lateral inner wall of the other orbit.

ABDOMINAL PERIMETER

In the section for abdominal perimeter measurement, the spine should be posterior and the umbilical part of the portal vein anterior.

Reporting

These are the parameters to be mentioned in the report. The list might appear too long but it is simple and one should routinely evaluate all these parameters.

Parameters to be routinely evaluated are mentioned as (R) and ones to be specifically looked in particular conditions are mentioned as (S).

FROM 05-10 WEEKS

- Uterine size (R)
- Location of gestational sac (R)
- Number of gestational sacs (R)
- Size of gestational sac (R)
- Yolk sac (R)
- Size of yolk sac (R)
- Embryo/fetus size (R)
- Menstrual age (R)
- Cardiac activity (R)
- Heart rate (R)
- Fetal movements (R)
- Trophoblastic reaction (R)
- Internal os width (R)
- Length of cervix (R)
- Any uterine mass (R)
- Any adnexal mass (R)
- Corpus luteum (present/absent) (R)
- Corpus luteum vascularity (S)

FROM 10-14 WEEKS

- Placental site (R)
- Liquor amnii (R)
- Fetal crown rump length (R)
- Menstrual age (R)

- Fetal movements and cardiac activity (R)
- Any gross anomalies (R)
- Nuchal translucency (R)
- Ductus venosus flow (S)
- Internal os width (R)
- Length of cervix (R)
- Any uterine mass (R)
- Any adnexal mass (R)

FROM 14-22 WEEKS

- Placenta (R)
- Liquor amnii (R)
- Umbilical cord (R)
- Cervix (R)
- Lower segment (R)
- Myometrium (R)
- Adnexa (R)
- Nuchal skin thickness (S)
- Cerebellar transverse diameter (S)
- Cisterna magna depth (S)
- Width of body of lateral ventricle (S)
- Inter-hemispheric distance (S)
- Ratio of the width of body of lateral ventricle to inter-hemispheric distance (S)
- Ocular diameter (S)
- Interocular distance (S)
- Binocular distance (S)
- Biparietal diameter (R)
- Occipitofrontal distance (R)
- Head perimeter (R)
- Abdominal perimeter (R)
- Femoral length (R)

- Humeral length (S)
- Foot length (S)
- Fetal movements and cardiac activity (R)
- Ductus venosus flow velocity waveform (S)

FROM 22-28 WEEKS

- All parameters of 14-22 weeks except nuchal skin fold thickness (R) and (S)
- Umbilical artery and uterine artery flow velocity waveform (S)

FROM 28-41 WEEKS

- Placenta (R)
- Liquor amnii (R)
- Umbilical cord (R)
- Cervix (R)
- Lower segment (R)
- Myometrium (R)
- Adnexa (R)
- Biparietal diameter (R)
- Occipitofrontal distance (R)
- Head perimeter (R)
- Abdominal perimeter (R)
- Femoral length (R)
- Distal femoral epiphysis (R)
- Biophysical profile (S)
- Color Doppler arterial (Umbilical artery, middle cerebral artery, descending aorta and both maternal uterine arteries) (S)
- Color Doppler venous (Umbilical vein, inferior vena cava and ductus venosus) (S)

Schematic Analysis for Fetal Anomalies

EXTRA-FETAL EVALUATION

Placenta	Umbilical cord	Liquor amnii
Thickness	Number of vessels	Echotexture
Location	Origin and insertion	Quantity
Morphology	Masses	Amniotic bands
Focal masses	Length	

Cervix	Lower segment	Pelvis
Internal os	Thickness	Masses
Length serial evaluation		

FETAL EVALUATION

Choroid plexus	Cerebellum	Cisterna magna
Cysts	Cerebellar transverse diameter	Depth
Hydrocephalus	Superior and inferior cerebellar vermis	Posterior fossa cyst
Isolated dilatation	Communication between fourth ventricle and cisterna magna	
Orbits	Face	Nuchal skin
Hypo- and hypertelorism	Lips	Thickness
Lens	Nostrils	Septations
	Ear	

Spine	Heart	Thorax
Coronal	Situs	Diaphragm
Longitudinal	Size	Lung length
Axial	Rate	Lung echoes
Ossification	Rhythm	Ribs
Soft tissues	Cofiguration	Masses
	Connections	Cardiothoracic ratio

Abdomen	Skeleton	Biometry
Gastrointestinal	Cranium	Biparietal diameter
Hepatobiliary	Mandible	Occipitofrontal distance
Genitourinary	Clavicle	Head perimeter
Pancreas	Spine	Abdominal perimeter
Spleen	Extremities	Femoral length
		Humeral length

Fetal Abnormalities in Trisomy 21, 18 and 13

Organ system	Trisomy 21	Trisomy 18	Trisomy 13
Head and brain	Mild ventriculomegaly	Dolichocephaly Strawberry-shaped skull	Holoprosencephaly Agenesis of corpus callosum
		Large cisterna magna Choroid plexus cysts Agenesis of corpus callosum	Ventriculomegaly Enlarged cisterna magna Microcephaly
Facial	Flat face	Micrognathia Microphthalmia	Micrognathia Sloping forehead Cleft lip and/or palate Microphthalmia Hypotelorism
Neck	Thickened nuchal skin fold Cystic hygroma	Nuchal thickening	Nuchal thickening
Cardiac	Ventricular septal defect Atrial septal defects Atrioventricular canal Echogenic cardiac focus		Ventricular septal defect Atrial septal defect Dextrocardia Echogenic cardiac focus
Gastro-intestinal	Hyperechoic bowel Esophageal atresia Duodenal atresia	Diaphragmatic hernia Omphalocele	Omphalocele

Contd...

Contd...

Organ system	Trisomy 21	Trisomy 18	Trisomy 13
	Diaphragmatic hernia	Esophageal atresia	
Urogenital	Renal pyelectasis	Hydrone-phrosis, Horseshoe kidney	Renal cortical cysts Hydronephrosis Horseshoe kidney
Skeletal	Short femur and humerus Clinodactyly of fifth digit Widely spaced first and second toes Wide iliac angle	Clubfoot deformity Generalized arthrogryposis Clenched hands	Postaxial polydactyly Camptodactyly Overlapping digits
Hydrops/ cutaneous	Nonimmune hydrops		
Liquor amnii		Third trimester— polyhydramnios	Third trimester— hydramnios
Biometry		Second trimester—onset intrauterine growth retarda-tion	Second trimester—onset intrauterine growth retarda-tion
Doppler	Abnormal ductus venosus waveform	Abnormal ductus venosus waveform	Abnormal ductus venosus waveform

Fetal Abnormalities in Triploidy and Turner's Syndrome

Organ system	Triploidy	XO
Head and brain	Ventriculomegaly Agenesis of the corpus callosum Dandy-Walker malformation Holoprosencephaly	
Spine	Meningomyelocele	
Facial	Hypertelorism Microphthalmia Micrognathia	
Neck	Cystic hygroma	Large, septate, cystic hygroma
Thorax		Pleural effusions
Cardiac	Septal defects	Coarctation of the aorta
Gastrointestinal	Omphalocele	Ascites
Urogenital	Hydronephrosis	Horseshoe kidneys
Skeletal	Syndactyly of the third and fourth fingers Clubbed feet	Short femur
Hydrops		Severe lymphoedema of all the soft tissues
Placenta	Enlarged placenta or small, prematurely calcified placenta	
Liquor amnii	Oligohydramnios	
Biometry	Severe, early-onset, asymmetric intrauterine growth restriction (affecting the skeleton more than the head)	
Doppler	Abnormal umbilical artery Doppler waveform, showing a high-resistance pattern	

Fetal Abnormalities in Maternal Infections

Organ system	Cytomegalovirus	Rubella	Toxoplasmosis	Parvovirus
Head and brain	Ventriculomegaly Intracranial calcifications Microcephaly	Microcephaly	Ventriculomegaly Microcephaly Intracranial calcifications	
Facial		Cataracts Microphthalmia	Cataracts	
Cardiac	Cardiomegaly	Septal defects		Pericardial effusion
Gastrointestinal	Hyperechoic ascites Intrahepatic bowel ascites calcifications	Enlarged liver and spleen	Intrahepatic calcifications Hepatomegaly Ascites	Ascites
Hydrops	Hydrops			Hydrops
Placenta			Thickened placenta	Thickened placenta
Liquor amnii				Polyhydramnios
Biometry	Intrauterine growth restriction	Intrauterine growth restriction	Intrauterine growth restriction	

Index

A

Abdominal perimeter 83, 194
Abnormal fallopian tube 170
Abnormal vagina 170
Acrania 57, 95
Adenomyosis 144
Adenomyotic uterus 148
Adnexal mass 54, 55, 160
Agenesis of the corpus callosum 95
Amniotic bands 89
Amniotic fluid index assessment
    71, 113, 193
Anechoic cysts/cystic lesions 160
Anechoic or hypoechoic area 40
Anencephaly 58, 95
Ascites 107

B

Biophysical score 123
Bleeding per vaginum 49
Breech presentation 115

C

Cardiac situs 80
Cephalic presentation 115
Cerebellar transverse diameter 191
Cerebellum 193

Cerebral artery 127
Cervical disorders 170
Cervical lesions 173
Cervix 25, 74, 92
Choroid plexus 33, 77, 95
Cisterna magna 78, 191, 193
Cleft lip 103
Clubfoot deformity 107
Color Doppler evaluation 181
Complex cysts 160
Confirming ovulation 176
Congenital diaphragmatic hernia
    103
Corpus luteal flow 53
Cranial biometry 194
Crown rump length 27, 30
Cutaneous thickness 191
Cystic adenomatoid malformation
    103
Cystic degeneration 148
Cystic hygroma 58, 98

D

Dandy-Walker malformation 98
Dermoids 164
Descending aorta 128
Doppler ultrasound 123
Ductus venosus 129
Duodenal atresia 107

E

Embryo 21
Embryonic bradycardia 31
Endometrial cancer 151
Endometrial changes 187
Endometrial fluid 151
Endometrial hyperplasia 151
Endometrial motion 181
Endometrial polyps 151, 153
Endometriosis 160
Endometritis 151
Endometrium 135, 151, 176
Esophageal atresia 103
Extra-fetal evaluation 200

F

Fallopian tube 138
Femoral epiphysis 117
Fetal biometry 116
Fetal evaluation 200
Fetal surveillance 131
Fibroids 144
First trimester scan 62, 64
Folliculogenesis 140
Functional cysts 160

G

Gestational sac 19

H

Hematometra 150
Holoprosencephaly 95
Hyaline degeneration 147
Hydrocephalus 95
Hydrometrocolpos 149
Hydronephrosis 107

Hydroureteronephrosis 107
Hypoechoic area 39

I

Inferior vena cava 130
Intrauterine contraception devices
156, 157

K

Kyphoscoliosis 105

L

Large bowel 191
Liquor amnii 21, 69, 88

M

Maternal infections 207
Meningocele/encephalocele 95
Menstrual cycle 180, 187
early proliferative phase 180
late proliferative phase 180
luteal phase 181
Myometrium 138, 144
Myometrium and adnexa 74, 93

N

Nuchal skin 193
Nuchal skin fold 190
Nuchal translucency 33 59, 190,
193

O

Obstetric scanning 132
Obstruction 144

Orbital measurements 194
Ovarian neoplasms 165
Ovarian stromal blood flow 188
Ovarian vascularity 187
Ovaries 138
Ovary in anovulatory cycles 176

P

Parameters to be routinely evaluated
    from 05-10 weeks 196
    from 10-14 weeks 196
    from 14-22 weeks 197
    from 22-28 weeks 198
    from 28-41 weeks 198
Paraovarian cysts 160
Pericardial fluid 191
Placenta 66, 86
    echo pattern 69
    focal lesion 66, 86
    location 66
    retroplacental area 86
    thickness 66, 86
Pleural effusion 103
Polycystic kidneys 107
Polycystic ovaries 168
Pouch of Douglas 142, 170, 173

R

Renal pelvis 190

S

Sac/embryo growth 46
Section for cranial biometry 76
Simple ovarian follicular cyst 167
Single line endometrium 181

Small bowel 191
Solid ovarian masses 168
Spinal meningocele/meningomy-
    elocele 103
Spontaneous abortion 50
Steps for ultrasound examination
    12
Synechiae 151

T

Theca lutein cysts 160
Trisomy 21, 18 and 13 204
Trophoblastic reaction 21
Tubo-ovarian abscess 160
Turner's syndrome 205

U

Ultrasound machine 2
    external device 10
    front panel with all knobs 2
    monitor 2
    transducers 2
Umbilical artery 125
Umbilical cord 70, 92
Umbilical vein 126
Uterine arteries 123, 124
Uterine calcifications 144
Uterine vascularity 51
Uterus 19, 135

V

Ventricular atrium 190, 191

Y

Yolk sac 21